Reversin

*How Liver Disease Helped Me Restore My
Health, Find My Voice and Learn to Live My
Very Best Life*

*By
Susan R. Pryde*

ISBN: 978-1-957180-03-8

Dedication

To my husband Neil —your love and support go deeper than any words can convey. I adore the life we have built and the wonderful adventures we share. The years are speeding by. I love you.

To my children, Taylor and Doug, Nick (Taylor's husband, very much a chosen child of ours now), my grandson, Greyson, and the new little wee one on the way — I can't imagine not being around to continue watching you thrive and participate in all the goodness life offers. And I want to do it with gusto. You all make life so beautiful. All your support has been unbelievable.

To my friends and family, thank you for being with me on this journey and all that came before it, for the laughter, the joy, and the shared sorrows. I seriously have the best cheering section in the world.

Contents

Endorsement by C. Scott Swendsen, MD

Oh, that all patients were like Ms. Susan R. Pryde! I can take very little credit for her remarkable progress, but I was glad to have a front-row seat cheering her on. To watch someone go from having a fairly bleak outlook after a new diagnosis of cirrhosis of the liver to, at present, having no cirrhosis or severe fibrosis of the liver is truly remarkable. Her story is one of self-empowerment that is attainable for all. She's a beacon or roadmap for others looking for inspiration about how to respond to a disheartening medical diagnosis. Before we even met for the first time she was reading and learning what she could do to change the path she was on. Knowledge is power and she harnessed it with great effect. I recommend her story to you most strongly and hope that you, too, can be successful in living happily and healthily.

C. Scott Swendsen, MD, Board Certified Gastroenterologist
Associates in Gastroenterology in Colorado Springs, CO

Preface

"How much time do I have?" I asked my specialist in June of 2021. Dr. Swendsen informed me that I had cirrhosis of the liver. After results from a routine physical in January of 2021 sent me spiraling down a path of fear and the unknown, it took six months and what felt like a lifetime to hear my full diagnosis. There were several blood draws, ultrasounds, a special liver scan, an upper endoscopy, a bone density scan, and a specialist. I had never heard of fatty liver disease, or how it could lead to cirrhosis of the liver.

In late August 2020, my husband Neil, our boxer pup Penny, and I embarked on the journey of a lifetime. We sold our home and most of our worldly possessions and purchased a fifth wheel trailer. We then began our dream of living life on the open road. I kept my day job, working remotely full time. Neil retired in 2018. We were already managing our healthcare remotely due to the pandemic, which was a blessing in disguise for us. Labs and bloodwork were scheduled wherever we happened to be at the time. Unfortunately, some concerning test results came back after that first visit. My liver enzymes were elevated!

Nonalcoholic fatty liver disease (NAFLD) is a disease in which too much fat has accumulated in the liver. NAFLD is diagnosed if more than 5% or 10% of the liver contains fat. Nonalcoholic steatohepatitis (NASH) is a more severe form of NAFLD, where liver swelling and damage begins to occur. Cirrhosis is severe liver damage, including hardening scars and limitations to liver function, which can lead to liver cancer and liver failure.

In this book, I share my personal story after being blindsided by a diagnosis of NAFLD that had progressed to NASH and early cirrhosis of the liver. I will share how I learned to navigate back to a place of good health through proper nutrition, changed mindset, and good resources.

Fatty liver disease is something that was not on my radar, and I found this to be true in the many support groups I joined. Since my main platform of communication, in the beginning, had been Facebook, I searched and found several groups on NAFLD, cirrhosis, end-stage liver disease (ELD), and NASH. I began reading and interacting, often finding more questions, which led me to the desire to dig deeper for answers.

My goal in writing this book is to raise awareness and help others with the disease overcome the obstacles they face, and to help as many people as I can find their unique path to healing through nutrition, self-care, and the proactive use of medical care.

If you suspect you have liver disease, please do not wait to seek medical attention, and always be your own advocate. Speak up if something doesn't feel right.

I will take you through my journey from the diagnosis and what I did to ultimately heal my body, mind, and spirit, to share what worked for me to reverse cirrhosis of the liver.

May this help you to find what will work for YOU!

Love, Sue

Part One

BEFORE

Susan R. Pryde

Life Before Diagnosis

In the years leading up to my diagnosis, I was eating and drinking all the wrong things, and put on quite a few pounds. I considered walking to the mailbox exercise! A lot of exciting and some stressful things were happening in life. COVID-19 and all the upheaval of 2020 were hard on so many of us. I was 55 years old and 260 pounds.

As for the exciting things, my husband Neil and I were planning to live our dream of traveling the country in our fifth wheel trailer. Well, it happened! We sold our house and hit the road! It was kind of like being on a perpetual vacation at first. Yes, I was still working 40 hours per week remotely, but every night after work and on the weekends, it was exploration time! Exploration included patronizing the restaurants and pubs. Neil and I enjoyed meeting the locals and soaking up the atmosphere in new towns. I was not actively trying to lose weight at the time and was in the mindset that I deserved to have fun! I had worked hard all my life, and this was a new adventure, I wanted to experience it all. That October, we landed in a riverside campground, with a very resort-like feel. We were living the dream! I found myself not worrying about how I ate, and a few extra cocktails fit right into the equation.

My food and alcohol choices looked a lot like this with absolutely no thought of portion control:

- Breakfast – my favorite biscuit sandwich with sausage patty, American cheese, butter, and ketchup. I would often eat two of these.
- Lunch – a lunchmeat and American cheese sandwich with chips of some kind and I am certain there was something sugary for dessert of the prepackaged chocolatey kind.

- Dinner – most often fast food, I found I loved the patty melts and french fries at the little riverside pubs near our campground. If we did not eat out, I was eating something quick, or meals prepared with little nutrition in mind. For example, ribs with sugary sauce, and burgers on a white bun with onions cooked in butter.
- Snacks – ice cream, lots of ice cream, potato chips, cheesy crackers with squirt cheese or peanut butter.
- Alcohol – once or twice a week we would stop at a pub and I would have upwards of 4-6 drinks. Also, sometimes after work, it was fun to pour a glass of wine or walk down to the tiki bar and have a pina colada and enjoy the river view. It felt like I was on vacation!
- Late-night snacks – very often after a night out with alcohol, I would come home and eat whatever I could get my hands on. It could be leftovers, chips, candy, or all of it in one sitting.
- Fluid intake – mostly diet soft drinks, coffee with sugary creamers, and very little plain water.
- Exercise – sedentary – with occasional short walks or hikes.

Despite it all, in the back of my mind, I knew this couldn't go on forever. I was feeling overheated all the time, and even though we hiked and explored on evenings and weekends, I huffed and puffed and could not go as far as I wanted to.

My discouragement led to more snacking, as I tended to eat more when I was down on myself. My inner voice was very unkind. I would tell myself to stop it and resolve every morning to change, then by noon I was snacking and overeating again, only to wake up feeling guilty the next morning. At this point, I did not know my weight. I had not brought my scale with me on this new adventure, but I did know that my clothes were suddenly shrinking. Looking back, my behaviors were the perfect storm for liver disease in the form of fast foods, processed foods, and no self-awareness about portions at all. A recent study shows that fast foods are very much linked to liver damage: An excerpt from an article on January 13, 2023, by Megan Brooks on WebMD Health states, *"They found that people with obesity or diabetes who take in one-fifth or more of their daily calories from fast food had severely high levels of fat in their liver, compared with those who eat less or no fast food. The general population had moderate increases in liver fat when one-fifth or more of their diet was made up of fast food."*[1] I was not thinking along those lines at all.

I was a yo-yo dieter my entire adult life. As a child, I was called chubby or "husky." It seemed that every time I would begin to reach a healthier weight, I would almost immediately gain it back, weighing more than when I started dieting. It was so depressing and frustrating. I knew that I used food to soothe my emotions, and alcohol to ease my shyness in social situations. I was an emotional eater, and alcohol made me feel more social — liquid courage. I thought it was easier to be outgoing if I had a drink in my hand; that getting a buzz would lower my inhibitions and awkwardness. I also smoked on and off since my late teens, and after several attempts to quit, it finally stuck in August of 2016. I used my weight as an

---

[1] *1* "Fast-Food Fans May Face Liver Damage," accessed March 9, 2023, https://www.webmd.com/diet/news/20230113/fast-food-fans-may-face-liver-damage.

excuse to go back to smoking, because I always lost weight when I took up the habit once more. Not a sound practice.

My medical state prior to diagnosis put me on the verge of being on cholesterol and blood pressure medication. My triglycerides were always on the higher end, and I developed sleep apnea and went on a CPAP machine in 2019. I had been on thyroid medicine since 2006 when we learned I had hypothyroidism, and my dosage was rising along with my weight. I was also experiencing intermittent upper right quadrant abdominal pain.

I also have epilepsy, which has been controlled with meds since 2008, after having several grand-mal seizures, and I was plagued by migraines for many years, which were debilitating.

Poor dietary choices certainly contributed to the cirrhosis, but alcohol was a factor as well. I was not a daily drinker by any means, and while my liver disease was not specifically caused by alcohol, I do not want to discount the role it played in my overall health. Here is a tool that can help calculate the alcoholic liver disease/nonalcoholic fatty liver disease index (ANI): "*This calculator is intended for use by health care providers. The results should not be used alone to determine medical treatment. This tool is a statistical model and is not a substitute for an individual treatment plan developed by a health care provider with personal knowledge of a specific patient*". [2] As my specialist had stated, my cirrhosis was very much related to the whole of my weight and eating habits. For

---

[2] 2"The Alcoholic Liver Disease/Nonalcoholic Fatty Liver Disease Index (ANI) - Medical Professionals - Mayo Clinic," accessed March 9, 2023, https://www.mayoclinic.org/medical-professionals/transplant-medicine/calculators/the-alcoholic-liver-disease-nonalcoholic-fatty-liver-disease-index-ani/itt-20434726.

Susan R. Pryde

reference, my liver enzymes[3] were elevated. In January of 2021, my AST was 77 and ALT 106, (I did not know my weight then) and when retested in April of 2021 my AST was 84, and ALT 112, MCV 85, and I weighed 260 pounds. A new study shows that even moderate alcohol consumption can lead to cirrhosis of the liver: *"In middle-aged women, cirrhosis incidence increases with total alcohol intake, even at moderate levels of consumption. For a given weekly intake of alcohol, this excess incidence of cirrhosis is higher if consumption is usually without meals, or with daily drinking."* [4]

Looking back at my life prior to diagnosis, it is clear to me now that all signs led to a serious illness. I knew it deep down inside, and it kept me awake at night, worrying about my weight, my drinking, and my overall health. I would wake each day wanting to change, yet a few hours in, those worries were stuffed back into the corner of my mind in an endless cycle of worry, regret, and low self-esteem. I was stuck, and I needed a helping hand. It was time to open my eyes and address each unhealthy habit, and find my way to health.

---

[3] "Elevated Liver Enzymes - Mayo Clinic," accessed May 15, 2023, https://www.mayoclinic.org/symptoms/elevated-liver-enzymes/basics/definition/sym-20050830.

[4] 4Rachel F. Simpson et al., "Alcohol Drinking Patterns and Liver Cirrhosis Risk: Analysis of the Prospective UK Million Women Study," *The Lancet Public Health* 4, no. 1 (January 1, 2019): e41–48, https://doi.org/10.1016/S2468-2667(18)30230-5.

The Winding Road to Diagnosis

While in Western Arizona in December 2020, I scheduled a routine physical and labs. The results of the labs revealed elevated liver enzymes. I had the COVID virus in December of 2020 — what a New Year's gift, yay! My primary care physician advised me COVID-19 could elevate liver enzymes, and to re-test in three months.

Most of our friends and family who got it had very mild symptoms. Mine settled in the digestive tract. I had nausea and diarrhea, body aches and fever. I slept for the better part of the week. At that time, I had not heard of COVID-19 manifesting itself this way. More recent research shows that COVID-19 can cause fibrosis of the liver. I wondered why my illness settled in the digestive tract while everyone else I knew had respiratory issues, pneumonia, and severe coughing. A recent article stated *"...After entry into the human body through the respiratory tract, coronaviruses can lead to liver injury via several approaches, including ACE2/DPP4-mediated hepatocyte injury, immune-mediated liver injury, ischemia and hypoxia, thrombosis, and drug hepatotoxicity. The manifestations of liver injury involve abnormalities in liver function test and pathological examination."* [5] To paraphrase, once the coronavirus enters the body through breathing, it can harm the liver in different ways. It can damage liver cells by interacting with ACE2/DPP4 receptors, trigger an immune response that harms the liver, reduce the supply of oxygen and blood to the liver causing damage, lead to blood clots in the liver, and cause liver toxicity when certain drugs are used. We can see the

---

[5]"Frontiers | Potential Effects of Coronaviruses on the Liver: An Update," accessed March 9, 2023, https://www.frontiersin.org/articles/10.3389/fmed.2021.651 658/full.

Susan R. Pryde

effects of liver damage by doing tests to check if the liver is working properly and by examining liver tissue.

One of the stresses of our wonderful new life was figuring out the medical piece of the puzzle. We would no longer be near our trusted physician or facilities. We were moving about the country and figuring out medical care on the fly. I had our new healthcare plan figured out in theory, but never did I imagine we'd have to test it with such intensity right out of the gate. Would we be able to find a doctor who could see us? Would there be a specialist nearby? There were so many questions. Between the COVID-19 illness, and my brand-new liver problems, we had a challenge ahead of us. We had booked our travel plans approximately one year ahead of time, to make sure we had a good spot to land in each state we would visit. This was a bit of a challenge because some campgrounds had closed due to COVID-19. When it came to medical needs, we had to consider that we would be moving to another state shortly and had to plan accordingly.

We moved on to Texas in March of 2021, where I scheduled more blood work to re-test my liver enzyme levels. No good. They shipped me off for a more comprehensive hepatic panel and an ultrasound. I didn't know what to think but I was getting scared. The ultrasound showed increased hepatic echogenicity with severe hepatic steatosis, and my liver was mildly enlarged. My heart dropped. I had no idea what this meant. I was first told in a voicemail that I had NAFLD which included a long list of foods not to eat. According to the American Liver Foundation *"(NAFLD) is the build up of extra fat in liver cells that is not caused by alcohol. It is normal for the liver to contain some fat. However, if more than 5% – 10%*

10

percent of the liver's weight is fat, then it is called a fatty liver (steatosis)." [6]

My daughter and I joked together, "what's left, ice cubes?" I mean, my liver is chonky...what the heck?? Hepatic echogenicity means that the ultrasound picked up evidence of possible fat in the liver. Severe hepatic steatosis means that there appears to be severe inflammation in the liver. *"Some individuals with NAFLD can develop nonalcoholic steatohepatitis (NASH), an aggressive form of fatty liver disease, which is marked by liver inflammation and may progress to advanced scarring (cirrhosis) and liver failure. This damage is similar to the damage caused by heavy alcohol use."*[7]

So, in a nutshell, my chonky liver struggled to filter toxins. It would set the first task of getting rid of toxins before helping me lose weight. On top of this, it was taking up extra space that my lungs and other organs needed to help me function. Besides the extra 100-plus pounds my body was carrying, I did not have room to receive the oxygen flow when I would try to hike. I was huffing and puffing and discouraged, but I tried.

My fear grew. I called the doctor back after consulting Dr. Google, who convinced me that my days were truly numbered. The response I got was in a message on my health portal that said simply, you have severe scarring on your liver, you have NASH, and you need to find a specialist. So, I consulted Google. And my fear

---

[6] 6"Nonalcoholic Fatty Liver Disease (NAFLD) - American Liver Foundation," May 23, 2022, https://liverfoundation.org/liver-diseases/fatty-liver-disease/nonalcoholic-fatty-liver-disease-nafld/.

[7] 7"Nonalcoholic Fatty Liver Disease - Symptoms and Causes," Mayo Clinic, accessed March 9, 2023, https://www.mayoclinic.org/diseases-conditions/nonalcoholic-fatty-liver-disease/symptoms-causes/syc-20354567.

turned to terror. When I say I consulted Dr. Google, back then I had no idea what a reputable source meant. So, I would glom onto the first result that popped up, and often it would be horrible news. I have found that much of the information that I call Dr. Google is not true and can lead us down a path of despair and quite possibly worse off than before.

At this point, I had already realized some changes were in order. I ditched Dr. Google and began researching scientifically reputable sites like Mayo Clinic, American Liver Association, Livestrong, and Psychology Today. I joined every support group I could find on Facebook, yet still, my fear grew. I signed up for the Noom[8] weight loss program to help get my eating under control. I began to adjust to foods that do no harm and could heal my poor liver. This was on April 12, 2021.

I could not find a specialist in Texas, so we looked forward to our next stop, near Colorado Springs. Neil found me one (what a good boy). Before meeting my new specialist, they told me I needed a test called a FibroScan which would stage the level of fat and scarring. *"FibroScan Testing is a recently FDA-approved non-invasive diagnostic device used to measure liver scarring or fibrosis caused by a number of liver diseases. Similar to undergoing a conventional liver ultrasound exam, outpatient FibroScan testing is quick, painless, easy, and provides a non-surgical alternative to the traditional liver biopsy to assess liver damage.* [9] When we got to Colorado, I went for more labs and got my FibroScan on May 21,

---

[8] 8"Noom: Stop Dieting. Get Life-Long Results.," Noom, Inc., accessed March 9, 2023, https://www.noom.com.

[9] 9"What Is Fibroscan | Testing Preparation & Expectations," Associates in Gastroenterology, accessed March 9, 2023, https://agcosprings.com/procedures/fibroscan/.

2021. I couldn't imagine I'd hear anything worse. It was bad enough already, right?

Several weeks later (and already many pounds lighter thankfully) I finally met my specialist in mid-June. Before meeting him, I had seen the results of my FibroScan in my medical portal. I had researched this scan and I knew how to read it. I was with our daughter and grandson that day and I asked her if I should read it now or wait. We agreed to read. As my eyes scanned the results, my breathing stalled, a heaviness settled in my chest, and the screen blurred, making it difficult to read. It was like watching a train wreck. I didn't want to read any further, but I could not look away. I stood up slowly, and reached out for our four-month-old grandson who was lying nearby, hugged him to my chest, and rocked. I told him "Please, please promise me to keep your body healthy "as the tears began to flow. Our daughter was in the kitchen, and I walked with him into her line of vision. When she saw the look on my face, she quietly asked me to tell her the news. We all hugged and cried. I am so grateful I was not alone. Later that afternoon, when Neil picked me up, I told him in the car. It was then that reality struck all of us.

I met my specialist, Dr. Swendsen, the following week, June 15, 2021, and boy did we do good. I love him. He's a keeper. He delivered the news I knew was coming and I cried again but I had a two-page list of questions ready for him. What can I eat, am I doing this or that right, how long can I live? Neil was with me, thank God. He told us that based on the results of my FibroScan, the fat (steatosis) score, which is measured by what is called CAP was 276, grading me as S2, with about 34% to 66% fatty change. The liver stiffness (fibrosis/scarring) score, measured in kilopascals (kPa) was 14.5, with a fibrosis score of F4, meaning I had cirrhosis. He estimated that my liver function was approximately 15%-20%. Cirrhosis is often classified as either compensated or decompensated.

Mine was considered compensated, which meant that I was in the earlier stages, where symptoms are still mild. This was hard news to take in, but he sat with us for an hour and was compassionate and honest. And he was very happy with my progress in the two months that had passed since learning something was wrong, despite limited knowledge of how to proceed.

The goal was to continue to learn what I had to do to freeze this disease in place, halting its progression. I shared with Dr. Swendsen a complete list of all the foods I was eating, and what exercises I was doing, and he approved all the items. I told him I had immediately stopped all alcohol on April 12 and had dropped all processed foods and fast foods from my diet. I can't believe this now, but I asked him if he thought I could have a glass of wine now and then. The moment I said it, I felt an immediate shame reaction, like "really Susan, what's your biggest worry right now?" He remained compassionate and said the safest route is no alcohol at all. We also discussed supplements and agreed to avoid them as well.

I needed a new ultrasound and bloodwork in 3 months and a new FibroScan 6 months out. I was hopeful my next FibroScan would show regeneration. Having cirrhosis of the liver places us at a greater risk of hepatocellular carcinoma (HCC), or liver cancer. We would now need to screen via ultrasound every six months. He told us that the incidence of HCC in cirrhosis patients was cumulative, growing higher every year. Per an article in Medscape *"...and one third of all patients with cirrhosis will develop HCC. The incidence of HCC is 1%-8% per year in all patients with cirrhosis..."* [10]All in all, Neil and I were quite relieved to hear Dr. Swendsen say that I was doing amazing and definitely healing. He said I was the

---

[10] "Hepatocellular Carcinoma: 5 Things to Know," accessed May 15, 2023, https://www.medscape.com/viewarticle/925146.

poster child for what to do and that I should write a book or a blog, and he even asked me what I've been doing to lose weight and make so many changes. He eased our minds by saying that my efforts showed I could live a long and healthy life if I kept on this path, and liver disease would not be the cause of my demise. So, despite all this heavy news, I began to feel like I had a fighting chance. Determined to win, I knew I had to continue researching how to freeze the cirrhosis in place and halt the progression. I believed in my heart that I would be able to do this. Leaving Dr. Swensen's office, I felt like I could achieve the impossible. I was on my way back to health.

My next task was to have an upper endoscopy (EGD) and a bone density scan. *"An upper endoscopy, also called an upper gastrointestinal endoscopy, is a procedure used to visually examine your upper digestive system. This is done with the help of a tiny camera on the end of a long, flexible tube. A specialist in diseases of the digestive system (gastroenterologist) uses an endoscopy to diagnose and sometimes treat conditions that affect the upper part of the digestive system."*[11] The bone scan would check for osteoporosis. *"Osteoporosis is a common skeletal complication seen in patients with chronic liver disease. Osteoporosis is usually asymptomatic and, if untreated, can result in fractures and impaired quality of life."* [12]

Cirrhosis can lead to problems in the upper gastrointestinal tract that are dangerous and can be life-threatening. Specifically, they would be looking for esophageal varices. *"Esophageal varices are enlarged*

---

[11] [11]"Upper Endoscopy - Mayo Clinic," accessed March 9, 2023, https://www.mayoclinic.org/tests-procedures/endoscopy/about/pac-20395197.

[12] [12]Anitha Yadav and Elizabeth J. Carey, "Osteoporosis in Chronic Liver Disease," *Nutrition in Clinical Practice* 28, no. 1 (February 1, 2013): 52–64, https://doi.org/10.1177/0884533612470145.

Susan R. Pryde

veins in the esophagus, the tube that connects the throat and stomach. Esophageal varices most often happen in people with serious liver diseases "[13] Although my portal vein (*"The portal vein (PV) is the main vessel of the portal venous system (PVS), which drains the blood from the gastrointestinal tract, gallbladder, pancreas, and spleen to the liver."*) [14]looked good in my liver ultrasound, there was a chance of obstructed blood flow and enlarged veins in my esophagus. This can also lead to portal hypertension and ascites (fluid in the abdomen) or hepatic encephalopathy (ammonia build up in the brain) which can cause confusion and disorientation. These veins can leak or rupture. If any varices were found, they can band them during the EGD procedure, placing an elastic band on the area to tie off any bleeding veins. There is no warning when a vein is about to leak or rupture, so we needed to investigate.

I went for the EGD and bone scan in August of 2021, and both came back normal. I had no varices and no sign of osteoporosis. Once signs of these more serious symptoms of varices, ascites and hepatic encephalopathy appear, cirrhosis becomes decompensated, and can lead to end stage liver disease or liver failure, sometimes requiring a transplant in order to survive.

I did have a bit of an ulcer in the area near my esophagus and stomach, which was treated with about a month of proton pump inhibitor, a medication used for

---

[13] [13]"Esophageal Varices - Symptoms and Causes," Mayo Clinic, accessed March 9, 2023, https://www.mayoclinic.org/diseases-conditions/esophageal-varices/symptoms-causes/syc-20351538.
[14] Carolina Carneiro et al., "All about Portal Vein: A Pictorial Display to Anatomy, Variants and Physiopathology," *Insights into Imaging* 10 (December 2019), https://doi.org/10.1186/s13244-019-0716-8.

acid reflux, heartburn, and ulcers. Thankfully, these were the results we anticipated and hoped for. Because I had no sign of ascites, portal vein hypertension, or hepatic encephalopathy, my cirrhosis was considered compensated, which is good.

It had become clear to me over the months that my job was to continue to learn how to heal my body, becoming ever clearer to me that to do so, I would need to address all of it, my heart, my head, and my body. I would have to learn to be healthy all around. No longer could I rely on sheer luck to live a long and healthy life. I had to make the effort to address the reality of why I overate, drank to feel likable, and find out what foods and exercise my body required. My band-aids were no longer serving me.

Susan R. Pryde

What You Need to Know About Your First Specialist Appointment

Before I get to the nitty gritty of healing, it's important to know how to handle that first specialist appointment. It was overwhelming to me, so preparing in advance eased my fears. Reading the experience of others in my support groups helped ease my mind. A caring member in my first liver disease support group shared a list of questions which I have expanded upon below.

I needed to keep all my dates, paperwork, notes, and referrals together, so I bought an old fashioned 18-month planner. Having everything in one place helped to ease my anxiety. I didn't have to rely on an emotional memory because I had it written down. Emotional memories are linked to strong emotions. While emotions are natural and valid reactions to difficult news, relying solely on emotional memory can cloud judgement and hinder your decision making.

With all forms of liver disease, slowing or stopping the progression is very important. To do this, you need to live a healthy lifestyle by eating healthier, add more fresh foods and lean protein, reduce your intake of processed foods, sodium, and unhealthy fats. While removing alcohol from your diet is equally important, it is essential to seek medical support first. Anyone can experience delirium tremens and other life-threatening complications from suddenly stopping alcohol. So, consult with your doctor first before making this change. *"Heavy drinkers who suddenly decrease their alcohol consumption or abstain completely may experience alcohol withdrawal (AW). Signs and symptoms of AW can include, among others, mild to moderate tremors, irritability, anxiety, or agitation. The most severe manifestations of withdrawal*

include delirium tremens, hallucinations, and seizures. " [15]
Avoid unnecessary medication. Aim for a healthy weight, whether that is to lose, gain or maintain. Exercise as able. Get plenty of rest and try to avoid stress. All this will help protect your liver and slow/stop the progression of liver disease.

Take a loved one to the appointment – it helps to have another set of ears. I took my husband Neil, and if I faltered, he stepped in and asked the questions. Also take a pad of paper and that planner I mentioned. Write down the answers to all questions. I asked every single question on the list, and read off every item of food I was currently eating that was on my list. Dr. Swendsen answered every question.

Questions to ask your specialist:
- What can be done to slow/stop the progression?
- What over-the-counter medicine can I take for pain, allergies, etc.?
  - Acetaminophen (Tylenol), Ibuprofen, heartburn meds, etc.
- Are there any fluid or food limitations I should follow?
  - Increase or decrease water? This may depend on fluid retention.
  - Nutrition based on specific case, or underlying conditions.
- What additional tests do I need?
  - EGD: upper endoscopy examines esophagus and upper gi tract.
  - Colonoscopy: examines the lower gi tract.

---

[15] [15]Richard Saitz, "Introduction to Alcohol Withdrawal," *Alcohol Health and Research World* 22, no. 1 (1998): 5.

- o Bone density scan: check strength of bones.
- o Biopsy: gathers sample of liver tissue.
- What stage is my liver disease?
    - o Is there inflammation and fat in the liver, or is there fibrosis and scarring and to what degree?
- What is the cause?
    - o Excessive alcohol or drug use?
    - o Hepatitis B or C infection?
    - o Fatty liver: caused by obesity or diabetes?
- Am I compensated or decompensated?
    - o Compensated: no/minimal symptoms, liver functioning.
    - o Decompensated: symptomatic, liver struggling to function.
- Do I need to avoid using or being around household cleaners?
    - o Overexposure to these toxins can be harmful. Read warning labels carefully.
- Do you recommend any vitamins or supplements?
- Are there other health issues that need to be addressed?
- Do I need to be drained due to ascites and how often?
    - o If cirrhosis is decompensated, ascites is swelling of the abdomen, which requires draining or other procedures to resolve.
- What symptoms do I need to watch for, and which should I seek help for ASAP? These may include:
    - o Confusion
    - o Abdominal or chest pain.

- o Fever greater than 101F
- o Abdominal swelling that is new or suddenly becomes worse.
- o Rectal bleeding, vomiting blood, or blood in the urine.
- Can you check me for Alpha One Antitrypsin Deficiency (simple blood test)? [A protein deficiency that can harm the liver or lungs].
- Do I need to get Hep A/B vaccine?
- What is my MELD Score? [Model for end stage liver disease: this ranges from 6 to 40 and is based on the results from liver specific lab tests].

Also, I recommend taking a list of all the foods you are currently eating. Two months before meeting Dr. Swendsen, I had joined a weight loss program and was still learning what to eat. Learning of his take on my progress was very important. So I showed him my food list and put a check mark next to each good item, and a "NO" next to the ones to avoid.

Susan R. Pryde

Understanding Liver Disease Progression

When I learned that my liver was struggling, I realized how little I knew about this vital organ. I had heard of cirrhosis, but it was only in the context of alcoholism. The correlation between liver damage and other risk factors never crossed my mind, and I did not understand how important the liver's role was in our overall health. *"Unlike the lungs or heart, we cannot feel our liver working. Many people don't think about their liver unless or until there is something wrong with it. Your liver is an incredibly hard-working organ with more than 500 different vital functions. Only your brain has more functions than the liver. Many of the liver's functions are related to your metabolism. These metabolic functions allow you to convert food to energy, break down food to basic building blocks needed by your body and eliminate waste."*[16] The liver is our first line of defense in the breakdown of every toxin we encounter, whether we consume, inject, touch, or breathe it. The liver helps prevent the accumulation of waste products.

I am sharing a general model of liver disease progression below. Be aware that some doctors may grade the liver injury slightly differently, but this represents a common interpretation.

Liver disease progression

- Hepatitis: swelling of the liver due to inflammation. Inflammation is the body's natural response to injury and an important part of healing or immune response.[17]

---

[16] *16*"The Healthy Liver - American Liver Foundation," June 9, 2022, https://liverfoundation.org/about-your-liver/how-liver-diseases-progress/the-healthy-liver/.

[17] "Hepatitis (Inflammation) - American Liver Foundation."

- Fibrosis: scarring of the liver. When someone has liver disease, their liver enters into a very dangerous cycle. Persistent inflammation, or hepatitis, sends nonstop signals to repair cells to continue depositing collagen. The extra collagen stiffens around the tissue like it is supposed to in the healthy liver; but, instead of a signal being released to stop the inflammation and discard the extra collagen, the inflammation continues, and even more collagen is deposited, leading to more stiffening. This is how fibrosis develops. [18]

- Cirrhosis: severe scarring of the liver. The final stage of fibrosis. Cirrhosis is often categorized as either compensated or decompensated. Someone with compensated cirrhosis doesn't necessarily look or feel sick. Their symptoms of the disease may be mild or nonexistent even though the liver is severely scarred. Someone with decompensated cirrhosis will feel and appear sick as their liver is struggling to function. [19]

- Liver cancer: Liver cancer is cancer that begins in the cells of your liver. While several types of cancer can form in the liver,

[18] [18]"Fibrosis (Scarring) - American Liver Foundation," June 9, 2022, https://liverfoundation.org/about-your-liver/how-liver-diseases-progress/fibrosis-scarring/.

[19] [19]"Cirrhosis (Severe Scarring) - American Liver Foundation," June 9, 2022, https://liverfoundation.org/about-your-liver/how-liver-diseases-progress/cirrhosis-severe-scarring/.

the most common type of liver cancer is hepatocellular carcinoma, or HCC, which begins in the main type of liver cells (hepatocytes).[20]

- End stage liver disease (ESLD): liver damage is progressive, which means that over time (without diagnosis or successful treatment), it can lead to cirrhosis or end-stage liver disease (ESLD). ESLD is also known as chronic liver failure.[21]

-

Common causes of liver disease

- Viruses
- Genetics
- Autoimmune disease
- Excessive use of alcohol
- Poor diet and/or obesity
- Reactions to medications, street drugs, or toxic chemicals

Most liver diseases damage your liver in similar ways and for many the progression of liver disease looks the same regardless of the underlying disease.[22]

---

[20] [20]"Liver Cancer - American Liver Foundation," June 9, 2022, https://liverfoundation.org/about-your-liver/how-liver-diseases-progress/liver-cancer/.

[21] [21]"End Stage Liver Disease - American Liver Foundation," June 13, 2022, https://liverfoundation.org/about-your-liver/how-liver-diseases-progress/end-stage-liver-disease/.

[22] [22]"The Stages of Liver Disease - American Liver Foundation," June 8, 2022, https://liverfoundation.org/about-your-liver/how-liver-diseases-progress/.

The level of fat (steatosis) grading

- Normal: up to 5% of fat in liver.
- S1: less than 1/3 of liver affected by fatty change (11% to 33%).
- S2: between 1/3 and 2/3 of liver affected by fatty change (34% to 66%).
- S3: more than 2/3 of liver affected by fatty change (67%)[23]

The level of fibrosis (scarring/liver stiffness) grading

- F0 to F1: liver is normal.
- F2: liver has moderate scarring.
- F3: liver has severe scarring.
- F4: liver has cirrhosis. [24]

This brochure[25] from the Canadian Society of Intestinal Research is the most comprehensive visual guide to cirrhosis of the liver that I have seen.

---

[23] [23]"Understanding Your Liver Elastography (FibroScan®) Results | Memorial Sloan Kettering Cancer Center," accessed March 9, 2023, https://www.mskcc.org/cancer-care/patient-education/understanding-your-fibroscan-results.

[24] [24]"Understanding Your Liver Elastography (FibroScan®) Results | Memorial Sloan Kettering Cancer Center."

[25] GIS, "Your Liver & Cirrhosis Poster," *Gastrointestinal Society* (blog), accessed March 14, 2023, https://badgut.org/information-centre/multimedia/your-liver-cirrhosis/.

A Medical Perspective on Susan Pryde's Case –
By Dr. C. Scott Swendsen, MD

Ms. Pryde has permitted me to share the medical facts of her case. She was referred by her primary care physician to my office for a FibroScan given her history of suspected Non-Alcoholic Fatty Liver Disease (NAFLD) and ongoing elevated liver enzymes on routine blood tests on April 27, 2021. Elevated liver enzymes suggest liver injury and always warrant investigation. The purpose of the FibroScan is to assess for steatosis (fat in the liver) and fibrosis (scarring of the liver).

FibroScan is a very reliable validated test, especially for fibrosis. It can provide a wealth of information that formerly could only be obtained by a liver biopsy. Given the cost and risk of a liver biopsy, FibroScan is the preferred initial test.

NAFLD is a very common cause of liver injury estimated by studies to be present in about 25-34% of the adult population in the U.S. Unfortunately, up to 25% of people with NAFLD will progress to cirrhosis of the liver. Cirrhosis carries a high complication and mortality rate. The FibroScan performed by our office on May 21, 2021, showed a CAP (Controlled Attenuation Parameter), which measures fat in the liver, to be 276.

This indicates moderate steatosis, or that between 34-67% of her liver was fatty. This is very irritating to the liver. Normally there should be no fat or negligible amounts in the liver.

Most often the causes for fat in the liver are from being overweight, diet choices, genetics, alcohol use, and diabetes. The FibroScan also showed a shear wave stiffness of 14.5 kPa, indicating F4 fibrosis or cirrhosis. The FibroScan was high quality, and the results were felt to be reliable.

Cirrhosis is generally felt to be irreversible or minimally reversible. Fibrosis is graded F0-F4. F0 is no fibrosis, all the way to F4 fibrosis or cirrhosis. Once F4 fibrosis occurs, studies have shown that usually only 15-20% of your liver remains as functional liver and the rest is scar tissue. Alcohol use can cause the FibroScan score to be falsely elevated. The FibroScan result appropriately prompted a referral to me for a clinic visit.

On June 15, 2021, I met Ms. Pryde in the clinic for the first time. She was naturally unsettled about her new diagnosis, having not yet met with a physician to provide information, context, and prognostic information for her new diagnosis of cirrhosis. She had, however, already performed a lot of research on her own about what needed to be done to prevent the progression of her liver disease. She reported to me that she had already lost 42 lbs. by the time we met. Her weight at our first visit was 217 lbs., with a BMI of 35. She had had zero alcohol for 8 weeks. She reported that prior to our visits she would drink some wine and liquor, mostly one to two drinks per setting, but on occasion would have up to five drinks.

The recommended limit for a female is one drink per day. We discussed the natural course of cirrhosis and getting tests to better understand her prognosis and mitigate complications of cirrhosis. Her initial blood tests showed that thankfully her MELD score was 6, which indicates mild cirrhosis. Her liver enzymes on the blood work were also normal. This was surprising given that her liver enzymes were quite elevated in January 2021 (AST 77, ALT 106) and April 2021 (AST 84, ALT 112). Those lab tests were both about 2x-3x what they should be, confirming ongoing liver injury from the fat in the liver. I am unable to ascertain whether fat is in the liver from weight or alcohol, but her liver enzyme pattern suggested it was from the weight. The best way to obtain normal liver enzymes with fatty liver is to lose weight and stop drinking. She must have done both well for her liver tests to be normal.

An upper endoscopy in August of 2021 revealed acid reflux inflammation, but thankfully no evidence of complications from cirrhosis such as esophageal varices or portal hypertensive gastropathy. An ultrasound was performed that revealed no evidence of liver cancer, which is a common complication of cirrhosis.

Our next follow-up in the clinic occurred on September 14, 2021. By this time Ms. Pryde had lost 32 lbs. by our accounting, and 80 or so by hers. BMI was down to 29 (from 35 just 3 months earlier). She looked and felt so much better. I asked her about how she had achieved such success and she relayed to me how she had joined support groups, was eating much healthier, and actively walked and hiked. She introduced me to Noom, which is an online nutrition counseling service that teaches the psychology of eating, along with the basics of nutrition and weight loss.

She was on an excellent path, and I expected that with such great lifestyle changes, she would halt the cirrhosis progression and possibly even see some regression of the fibrosis score.

She was not satisfied with just losing the 5-10% weight recommended by studies to reverse the injury from NAFLD.

She was determined to keep going until she achieved a normal weight. Accordingly, we ordered a repeat FibroScan for January of 2022.

The repeat FibroScan showed that she had no significant steatosis and F0-F1 fibrosis! Her CAP score was 204, kPa was 3.8. This result almost felt unbelievable, but the quality control parameters on the test again showed it to be an accurate, reliable test. This result confirmed that she no longer had cirrhosis, and in fact had almost no fibrosis at all. This was an objective testament to the power of healthy choices.

Our final clinic visit together was in February of 2022. At that visit, she weighed in at 149 lbs., with a normal BMI of 24. This comes to a total objective weight loss of 68 lbs. since we met. This office visit felt more like a victory lap than anything else. One more FibroScan is ordered for early 2023 for extra verification of our findings.

C. Scott Swendsen, MD

Part Two

HEART

Honesty and Well-Being

I have had many "I know I need to do this" moments in my life. I have successfully navigated doing them to some degree several times, but each time I was able to convince myself that continuing was no longer necessary or I'd gotten too cocky and derailed thinking "I'll just continue tomorrow or later today". The next thing I knew, a year passed (or seven). Where am I going with this? Well, there came a day when I had to face all the little lies that I told myself. When I learned something might be wrong, at first I tried to say, "oh it's nothing, the doctors got this wrong, I feel pretty good for the shape I'm in, so it can't be true, right?"

Self-care is extremely important to one's general well-being. We all know what we should do, right? Tell the truth. Simple. Well, somehow, it's not always so simple when we are talking to ourselves. And it's especially challenging when facing difficult situations; times where it may be easier to suppress the honest reality, soften it and brush by it for another day.

Most of us can relate to this in the form of weight loss. I mean we all start the week, day, and meal off with good intentions when we decide "the time is now!" But how easy is it to get derailed? One brownie set within a hundred yards, and soon we are running to gobble it up and left wondering what the heck just happened. Medical? Yeah, that one's a kicker, too. How often do we experience certain emotions but conveniently fail to communicate them to our doctor due to embarrassment? Well, here's the thing: If we're not ready to face the truth, then we're not ready to make a change. We become skilled at deceiving ourselves by ignoring or justifying the things we know we should be doing. By disregarding our body's signals and convincing ourselves that everything is fine, we give ourselves permission to carry on with our daily lives without fearing the consequences. Personally, I would avoid visiting the doctor because I knew I would have to step on the dreaded scale. There were times when I hadn't weighed myself, and I definitely didn't want my doctor to once again inform me that I needed to lose weight.

I had pain in the right side of my chest on and off like a knife for several years. I told the doc about it once, thought it was anxiety, and didn't want to face what else it might be. While it hurt enough for me to make an appointment, I downplayed it once I was on the examination table. I can honestly say looking back, that I really did not want to hear what might be wrong with me, which resulted in me never going back to re-investigate. I didn't go even when the pain behind my breast would arrive in the middle of the night, a heavy pressure that would awaken me in a cold sweat, scared I was having a heart attack, or thinking maybe I had breast cancer! But I would breathe deep and try to clear my mind and come morning, sweep it under the rug. I didn't know at the time, that the liver has no pain receptors, but the casing around it and any organs an inflamed/enlarged liver presses on will hurt. I was feeling that pressure. The liver is more the boss than I realized, friends. As I mentioned previously, mine measured 17cm in March of 2021, and it was super angry. According to an article from Stanford Medicine *"...the liver span at midclavicular line is normally 6-12cm."*[26] This can vary based on age, sex, and weight.

I didn't go in when I was having bloating and diarrhea after heavy, unhealthy meals, or a night out drinking wine with friends. The morning after such nights out, I spent in the bathroom, my body trying to rid itself of the alcohol and food until mid-day. I lived on Imodium

---

[26] [26]Evangelos Kalaitzakis, "Gastrointestinal Dysfunction in Liver Cirrhosis," *World Journal of Gastroenterology : WJG* 20, no. 40 (October 10, 2014): 14686, https://doi.org/10.3748/wjg.v20.i40.14686.

those days. Without it, I couldn't be more than 100 yards from the bathroom. *"GI symptoms are common in cirrhotics compared to healthy controls. Overall, up to 80% of patients with cirrhosis have been reported to have one or more relevant GI symptom. The most common GI symptoms reported include abdominal bloating in 49.5% of patients, abdominal pain in 24%, belching in 18.7%, diarrhea in 13.3%, and constipation in 8%"* [27] Yeah, super embarrassing. Symptom of the liver not processing foods, right? Bingo! Tell anyone about it? Heck no! For me, drinking went hand in hand with eating improperly. Once I had a few drinks, thoughts of staying on track with my diet went straight out the window. In fact, I could easily consume a second dinner and two extra desserts after coming home from a party or a night out with friends. I just didn't care on those nights. I would wake up in the morning feeling so depressed and disappointed in myself, and inevitably I had gained back the few pounds I had lost that week in one single evening. This set me in a horrible cycle of losing weight during the week, only to gain it back on a Saturday night. The next day, feeling down on myself, I would eat horribly all day, reasoning that I had already messed up my diet for the week, I might as well have fun! Bring on the greasy cheeseburgers, french fries, pizza, and ice cream. What the heck?

I had swelling in my lower legs, and hands, mostly when I woke up in the mornings. I also injured my left knee in 2019 and wore a brace for approximately nine months, having torn my MCL and cracked a bone in the knee. I attributed much of my weight gain to this lack of mobility and blamed much of my swelling on this. I reasoned that I could not move as much, so of course it made sense. Looking back at photos of myself I see also how swollen my face was, and how horribly I snored, leading me to a diagnosis of sleep apnea, and treatment

---

[27] [27]Kalaitzakis.

Susan R. Pryde

with a CPAP machine. "*A CPAP (continuous positive airway pressure) machine is one of the most common treatments for sleep apnea. It keeps your airways open while you sleep so you can receive the oxygen you need for optimal function. CPAP machines can significantly improve sleep quality and reduce your risk for a number of health issues, including heart disease and stroke.*"[28] I can now see the connection of the extra fluids I was retaining, and the inflammation that ran through my entire body.

I experienced a severe intolerance to heat for several years. I thought, "Susan, you're just too overweight, lose weight and you'll be fine." I never considered that when the liver is not functioning well, it's overworked and it overheats. Thus, I lost the ability to keep cool, or regulate my body temperature. I was experiencing night sweats as well. It seemed that everyone around me was cool as a cucumber while I was red faced and so hot I didn't know what to do with myself.

I was aware the last few doctors' visits revealed my cholesterol, triglycerides and blood pressure were reaching the levels that would put me over the edge to needing medication to bring them down. I did not want to take more medications, so I solved it by not going back to the doctor. If I was unaware of a problem, then I didn't have to fix it, right? In my head, all of this could be solved by losing weight. "That was all that was wrong with me" I reasoned. Had I not brushed off those symptoms, and dug a little deeper, maybe, just maybe, I would have caught this before it tipped to cirrhosis.

So, when I initially heard I may have NAFLD, and had no idea what that was, my first thought was, ok, lose the weight, girl. And that alone scared me. I still didn't

---

[28] [28]"CPAP Machine: What It Is, How It Works, Pros & Cons," Cleveland Clinic, accessed March 9, 2023, https://my.clevelandclinic.org/health/treatments/22043-cpap-machine.

know the full diagnosis, but I had found Dr. Google, and learned that NAFLD was bad enough. I am so glad I looked in the mirror at that moment and said enough is enough.

I was starting to realize that if I did nothing, I could end up getting cirrhosis and liver failure, and possibly end up on a transplant list. Little did I know that I was already at cirrhosis, which is stage 1 liver failure.

Listen to your body and get in tune with its message. Hopefully, all is well, but what if it isn't? Stop sweeping stuff under the rug, or something minor could grow into something frightening. I did not know that the liver is like your car's engine, regulating so many of the body's functions. I can tell you that all my symptoms seemed unrelated; but boy they were very connected. Hindsight is crystal clear. Liver disease is most often a very silent issue until it's too late. Don't wait until it is too late, no matter what the problem may be. And here is where my self-growth was born. I needed to begin cultivating my self-respect and turn inward for the answers I needed to heal. You can do the same.

Susan R. Pryde

Taming the Dragon

One of my dear family members told me I was like a warrior princess in my healing effort. I imagined I was slaying my dragon within. Or rather, taming it. I needed it, you see, to behave in the manner for which it was created. It required my love.

I was so lost in the beginning on what it would take to heal my liver. I could not fathom what it would look like to heal, or even if I could. Who could I turn to that had the answers? All I knew was it felt like my body had betrayed me. I was going along living life, and this tap on my shoulder came, and it was my liver back there saying. "Hey, hold up. We need to talk." My first view of this liver wasn't pretty. I saw it as a foreign object, dead set on taking me out of this life, a dragon with a hearty flame indeed. When I turned to face it, I could feel the heat, and see the smoke curling from its nostrils while it chuckled at me, "what are you going to do now?" it seemed to say. To say that I screamed and fainted would be an understatement. I didn't expect to awaken unburnt; heck I didn't expect to awaken at all! My gut reaction was to start chopping away at the pain it caused. Chop away I did! I slashed wildly at it for a few months, cutting calories here, dumping the alcohol there, slicing away the white bread. I was also hacking away my self-worth because, after all, I had done this to myself, right?

At some point, the dust settled, and I stood panting, sword in hand. The frenzy of fear had quieted, and I blinked, looking around. The landscape looked different somehow. There were things I hadn't noticed before in my path — light and beauty, and hope. I realized that now that I had cut out all the damaged pieces, it was time to find new and better parts to replace them with. I could not literally "slay" everything that I was, I needed to tame and refine the best parts of me, and allow them room to grow.

I realized I had to look back to where my self-care lost its footing. My father passed away when I was eight, three days after my birthday, on Father's Day. I was a daddy's girl. He took me for walks outdoors, he would let me go barefoot, and he loved camping and boating and nature. The morning he died, I had awakened from a dream of me running along the beach while he floated up and away and out of sight. I recall running into my parents' room and crying, telling him not to leave me. He soothed me and held me and said he would never leave me. That morning we were taking the canoe that he had hand-made on its maiden voyage. My mom was afraid of water, so he alternated taking my brother and me out. I went first. He returned with me and took my brother, but this time the canoe tipped.

My brother had a life jacket on, but dad did not. I could hear dad saying it would be ok. I was on the beach watching it all unfold with my mother. I had no shoes on, and I ran as fast as I could over the rocks and sand to reach a nearby building for help. When I returned, the kind people I found took their boat out to help retrieve dad and my brother while mom and I waited. As they towed the boat and the two of them back to shore, dad was lying on his back with his knees up in the bottom of their boat. A woman's hands that were not my mother's had encircled my shoulders from behind. She had long brightly colored nails, and she was holding onto me tight. I don't remember what anybody was saying, I only recall a feeling of dread. My father drowned that day, and it was too much for my eight-year-old brain to comprehend.

This was the day my innocence died. The day I found out that things don't always turn out happily ever after. This was the day I first tasted grief and it has been sitting in a ball deep down inside ever since, internalized. Losing my dad affected so many aspects of my growth over the years. My mom closed the door to friendship on that day. She rarely let others in, so afraid she would lose them like she had the love of her life. She loved my brother and me very much, but she was no longer demonstrative. She held back so many feelings, and so many things a child needs from a mom to grow into a healthy emotional adult. She was a wonderful woman, yet she was forever heartbroken. I look back and I know now that deep down inside I understood that she had all she could handle in her own emotions, and I needed to deal with my own.

My dragon was the grief in my belly. I didn't identify it; rather I danced around it and ignored it; stuffed it down in a vault. Our family dynamic was still good, we loved each other, mom, brother, and I, but we were a very small nucleus. I looked up to my brother, strong, smart, and successful in school. I tended to be the small quiet girl in his circle of friends. I was more like a mascot in their lives, but they all treated me well and I felt safe and loved. I had a few good girlfriends, but I was awkward with the boys, not knowing how to act around them. I'd lost the best one, after all. I lost the one I admired most.

When I met Neil in the fall of 1983, I realized my days of running from relationships with men were coming to an end. Neil was fun, carefree and came from a rowdy, loving family. The youngest of four, he was living life out loud. His parents had moved to Las Vegas earlier that year. His two brothers were off in the Air Force, while he and his sister were living in a town not far from mine. We met through mutual friends and at first, I thought "what a great guy! He's so much fun and he's a great friend!" but he kept showing up where I was.

Back then I had a horse, and I spent hours at the barn, out on the trail or in the arena, exercising her. I would come out to my car and find a rose and a note from him under my windshield. I was out on a date one night with another guy and we stopped at a local place I liked to

38

go with my friends and Neil showed up. I recall he was quiet and seemed sad. I told my date it was time for him to go, it was our first time out and my friend was sad! My friend was more important than some guy I hardly knew. So, I sat down next to Neil, and I asked him what was wrong. It turns out he liked me, and I mean LIKED me, and not as a friend. What? This was shocking! I had never considered it before. So, I gave him my phone number and said, "call me." He did, and we have been together since that day, currently married over 35 years and still going strong. Neil is the reason I was able to begin opening my heart again to love. I am still grateful for him every day. By the way, the guest check with my phone number is still in his wallet, laminated. Cool, eh?

My dragon thrived, smoldering in the form of eating for comfort, drinking for confidence, and low self-esteem. I now know that the food and the alcohol held my self-esteem down in the dungeon. They were hurting me deeper than I knew. The day I found out I had cirrhosis was the day that bubble popped. This was the day I knew that I had to face my reality, choose to live for myself and live the right way. I couldn't properly love my husband, children, grandchild, and friends if I had no love for myself. I needed to tend to the good in me and earn my own self-respect and love. I needed to learn to trust myself and my own decisions and have a healthy heart, one strong enough to heal my body.

I am taming the dragon that lived in my belly by allowing myself to experience my emotions. It was never my enemy; it required a voice and a lot of compassion. I must allow myself the grace to feel and address all that makes me alive to keep it tame and be whole.

Susan R. Pryde

Self-Care

How often in life do we neglect our own self care? As the universe often does, it set things in our path that related to what we needed on a given day. I had noticed this occurring quite a lot suddenly. Early on in my healing, my Noom lessons covered this subject, placing it squarely in front of me with perfect timing. I love how this works! According to an article in Psychology Today *"Self-care involves nurturing your body, mind, and spirit. It's about replenishing ourselves. Each person has their own idea of what self-care means to them and what activities are personally nurturing."*[29]

For the first time that I can recall I addressed each aspect of self-care. Not a little bit, but a LOT of bits. 100% on board. I never realized how intertwined the body, mind, and spirit are to the health of my whole being. Joy grew joy, gratefulness bred gratefulness, and anger brewed more anger. Well, you get the drift. Whatever you emulate, grows. Stress was a big one; any negative energy for that matter. It was so hard on the body. It was downright damaging in fact. My specialist told me to try to stay out of stressful situations. Then we laughed. But oh, it was true. To do this, I had to be willing to purposefully seek positive ways of loving my life, which looks different to all of us.

There were several things that helped me reduce stress in my life. I formed emotional connections with loved ones, and was present and engaged in those interactions. I spent time in nature, where I saw and experienced all the critters, flora, fauna, breeze, and

---

[29] [29]"14 Self-Care Rituals to Practice Now | Psychology Today," accessed March 18, 2023, https://www.psychologytoday.com/us/blog/the-empowerment-diary/202207/14-self-care-rituals-practice-now.

colors. Whenever things went south, I would take five minutes to close my eyes and breathe. I worked on becoming and staying grounded, seeking out humor in situations rather than frustration. I made sure to take time out for activities that brought me joy. For example, while we could see some grand sites from behind the windshield, I enjoyed immersing myself in nature and using my own two feet. Being a camera nerd, I would set my camera to "sports" mode and capture stuff flying by the window when we were driving. I loved zooming in on intimate close-up shots of living beings. Those critters may not have appreciated the noise of that vehicle disturbing their day, so I needed to be able to use my feet.

I wasn't always sunshine and roses. I got sad, I feared for a long time that it was a little too late to heal, and I became frustrated and even lonely. But each time one of those feelings surfaced I tried to make a distraction either in my head or body. I could not hide in a bubble. I had to feel the feelings, find my way through them, acknowledge them, and move on. I meant to live fully, joyfully, and positively.

I suddenly began to BELIEVE in myself and the power I had over my surroundings, my attitude, my health, and my life. I was a work in progress, a sculptor, a student, an observer, and a lover. I discovered a love of poetry. Surrounding myself with things I loved was important in developing my self-care. I stumbled across Mary Oliver's work when I first began working poetry into my routine. The poem called *Invitation* spoke to me loud and clear. I realized I was missing a deep connection in my life with people, things I loved doing, and the outdoors. I was rushing through life skimming the top. I realized how much I needed to make changes in my life and this poem smacked me between the eyes, I felt the call to action to take charge of my own life.

What will it take to get you to a place where you feel worthy of taking care of yourself? What is holding you back? Don't you realize, beautiful soul, that your family deserves to have you whole and healthy for as long as possible? Your presence here is very much needed. If not an unworthiness, what is the feeling that makes you hurt yourself so, are you conscience of it? I want you to really think about this. Take the time to dig deep. What small admission can you own today that you are willing to make a tiny change?

Make one little change to make and hold fast. Once you do that, another tiny one, then another, and another until one day, you turn around and see a huge pile of changes, bigger than you ever could have dreamed had you tried to address them all at once. This isn't a race; let every change take you higher. Place the new foundation, step up on it, and place another. If it cracks, fix it, and move on, figure out why it didn't sustain. Each step will take a different effort, more or less time, let it. It's ok. Be proud of each one. Let yourself feel them, more and more as you go. Stop allowing excuses.

Feeding the Spirit

Something that became ever so important to my self-care was the idea of living in full right now. I learned to give myself permission to seek out people, places, and activities that lit my fire. I made time for the good stuff. The time was now, to listen to my intuition more and to follow where my heart led.

It is important to engage in activities that make us feel alive. For me this meant time with family and friends. I wanted to BE a better friend, one who was paying attention and truly there for others. Holding that grandbaby for hours on end until he squirmed, or his parents pried him out of my arms. It meant taking long walks in nature and holding hands with my sweetie. Taking time to photograph all the beauty I saw around me. Creating art from a favorite photo or place. It may have been singing harmonies with a friend, or alone in the shower. Delving down deep into whatever I was doing, feeling, studying, touching, or learning. Allowing the wonder and joy that is life to plant its seed in my heart. Living, in all its glory, pain, sorrow, and joy is such a beautiful thing.

Let the sun dazzle me! I allowed myself to be distracted by the buzz of the bee or startled by the brush of the flower along the path. I wanted to stop and gaze, smell, and feel all that beauty had to share with me. It was during those times that the weight of worry lifted from my shoulders, lightened my heart, and cleared my head. It was then that I became the most in love with life and learned how worth living life truly was. Engaging in all those activities helped me to face whatever challenge awaited me.

Did you know a grizzly bear has a heart-shaped face? I discovered this one day while searching for some candy for my soul. We all know nutrition is important, but it's not always something to ingest. Usually, when I created a full-blown color portrait, I first sketched out the subject in my artist's journal. I kept a sketch of every piece that I created in the journal with the date it was drawn, the type of animal it was, its name along with its owner's name. Often, I would create portraits of pets for friends and acquaintances. For this grizzly, I opened the reference photo on my phone, and I ran my finger along the lines of her face. I realized the basic shape of her face was a heart, with big round, fluffy ears. This path I've been on is so much about following my heart that it struck me as a fitting subject to draw next. I knew that it was time to incorporate art back into my life.

Now that comfort food or a glass of wine is off the table, I turn to other fulfilling activities to lift my spirits. I had always been a positive person, but there were so many changes, I found myself sad and overwhelmed. Spending so many hours learning to improve my health was draining and took a lot of mental effort. The research paid off, though, and I enjoyed excellent progress. I have achieved better health than I thought possible, enjoying tons of new energy. I even had some cute new clothes. I felt younger and so much healthier, but it was important to make time for quiet activities that I adored. I needed to spend time doing things where I could forget my worries and my studies for a while.

I love creating art, reading, and learning, and I found that I had set those things aside for months. Finally, about 10 months in after diagnosis, I realized it was time to bring some of the joy back into my life. I unearthed my treasure trove of art supplies I had stored away and set them up in the fresh air. I took over the entire picnic table and got a little lost working on drawing a horse, my favorite animal. My love affair with horses goes way back. I started drawing them in kindergarten as soon as I learned to hold a pencil. I would sit with my spiral bound notebook and draw horse after horse, hoping the teacher wouldn't catch me. I don't think she ever did. I don't recall it, anyway. I was lucky through the years to have art classes available to me in school, and I kept at it.

I'm quite sure I purchased every book I could find on drawing animals. I took a few college-level classes and community art classes. I loved to paint in oils and watercolor, or charcoals. Creating art was much like reading a good book to me. I could get lost in the piece, and when I came back to earth, POOF, there was something beautiful on the canvas. I had taken a few decades off from art while raising children. Don't we always set aside these types of things as a parent? It seemed selfish in my mind to ignore the kids and draw.

I can tell you now, it would not have been selfish in the least. I could have drawn with them, but hindsight is always clear. I switched to a less messy form of art a few years before we hit the road in our fifth wheel. I knew we would not have the space for many extras, but I made room for colored pencils, pastels, charcoals, and good-quality paper. All these are portable and not too messy. I try to fit time in to create whenever I can, and often from the photographs I have taken on our hikes.

I've learned to be ok with whatever signals my body and mind are sending me. Play when the energy is high, research when the brain is curious, and rest when the body or mind is weary. Seek out the things that nurture and make the heart happy.

Walking in nature with Neil, our sweet pup Penny, and a camera helped me to lay the foundation for feeding my spirit. When I got out in nature, I came home with a sense of quiet confidence, and a loaded camera. I was feeding my creative side in the form of art. Combining my love of critters, colors, and movement together helped to trick me into exercising just a little bit more. I saw this as a win-win.

Susan R. Pryde

It is so very important to fill our lives with beauty and wonder, whatever that may look like for us. If something sounds interesting, it is very much worth our effort to give it a try. I don't want to wake up one day and say "Ok, I'm done. I don't want to work this hard for my health anymore, pass me the bacon. I'm going to sit in this chair the rest of my life" (which would be much shorter). I intend to hold on to this healing I have worked so long and hard for.

Somehow, this terrible diagnosis put me in tune with how I was supposed to be living. I was no longer mad at myself or disappointed I didn't get it until after illness struck. I was grateful it appeared in time for me to rise. I was happy doing the things that fed my spirit. Even as I write this my thought is "I'm living my dream writing these words right now, I'm following through, not just thinking about doing it, and it's amazing!" It would thrill me if just one reader gets the fire to help themself because they read something here — something that clicked in them to find inspiration and better health. This, right here, would make my day.

Support and Human Connection

Life finds ways to grow in unexpected places. The mental side of healing is equally important as the physical. Allowing others to be there for me, and not do it all alone was difficult at first. As I became stronger in the self-care area, I grew less shy and began to speak up more. I became better at giving myself to others and being able to receive what others had to offer. I realized it was too painful to suffer in silence. I needed warmth and love and the encouragement of others to help build my strength and resolve. It's easy to get trapped in a tangled web of fear, loneliness, and confusion.

> *"Loneliness and social isolation may be among the worst aspects of any chronic illness. More than 50% of Americans are socially isolated regardless of where they live or the size of the town or city."* [30]

I shared earlier about my husband, Neil. We have been through lots of things together, as all couples have. Neil has had to navigate how to care for a wife who has done a 180 in so many ways. He suddenly had a wife full of fear, frustration, dietary changes, and doctors' appointments. He also had to face his own fears of dealing with a sick spouse, a bit of a double whammy. It wasn't lost on me that I wasn't the only one trying to re-map this life. I'm sure I was not always easy to deal with, but he never complained. In my head, I always thought about how hard it must be for him, and this brought feelings of guilt on my part. We could no longer be the carefree,

---

[30] [30]"Heal by Connecting with Others | Psychology Today," accessed March 9, 2023, https://www.psychologytoday.com/us/blog/anxiety-another-name-pain/202205/heal-connecting-others.

couple — I was holding us back. Now we had to stop and think about where we were going and plan ahead as much as possible.

Neil helped me to step outside of my comfort zone and rebuild the best parts of our life together. We simply had to find better restaurants, for one! If an option was not available, he is an amazing cook and has learned how to prepare liver-friendly meals (they are superior to most restaurant food, anyway). He took an interest in what I needed and came through with delicious seasoning, minus all the sugar, extra sodium, and unhealthy fats. Neil listens to my fears or anxieties and comes up with ways to soften them. He sat with me at my appointments and participated. He encourages me to keep going every single day. He walks with me. He talks things out with me. He balances me. And now, while I'm writing this book, he's patient while I am yet again, distracted. In the face of struggle, we need that go-to person. Whether a spouse or a very trusted friend, we need someone who has our back and can help us by being strong when we are not. I owe you one, baby!

During my healing process, I came to realize the true importance of friendship. It's easy to get caught up in the day-to-day busyness and let long gaps in connection occur. At first, I was hesitant to burden anyone with my struggles. I was still working on my self-worth and questioned why anyone would want to hear about my challenges. However, I soon realized that this belief couldn't be further from the truth. Taking the brave step to reach out to close friends and family, I made an effort to connect with them through phone calls. Hearing their voices and sharing emotions became essential. I understood that the written word alone could be difficult to decipher, especially given the circumstances. Opening up to others brought a tremendous sense of relief as I received warm and caring support. While there were many questions, they actually helped me approach things calmly and think them through. I no longer felt like I was spinning my internal wheels; I had the valuable input of others to guide my thoughts.

In the past, I used to only share the happy side of myself with my friends, fearing that I would burden them. However, I've come to understand that seeking a deeper connection with loved ones means sharing both joy and sorrow. It's one of life's greatest gifts. Over time, I have become more authentic, allowing myself to express genuine emotions when interacting with others. I am fortunate to have some incredible friends, and I strive to reciprocate the support they have shown me.

The other piece of making connections has been finding others with liver disease. Sharing common issues can help us feel understood, and less alone in our struggles. I didn't know anyone in my immediate circle who had liver disease. The connections I have made with this new tribe of liver warriors are strong. We can ask tough questions and share findings together. Knowing how others deal with things can ease our worry or provide insight when escalation to a medical team is the way to go.

In life, there are countless moments when we need the support and care of others. It's not only about receiving advice or guidance but also about sharing wisdom, laughter, and finding a lighter perspective when we take things too seriously. Providing this kind of support to our friends is equally important. When a friend is going through a difficult time, I have found myself reaching out and asking, "Do you need someone to listen or would you like a distraction?" I am ready to offer either one. While I have always cherished my friendships, I am actively working on being more present and less distracted when we spend time together. Being fully present means engaging my senses, opening my heart, and giving my undivided attention instead of constantly searching for what I will say next. I am realizing that listening is an art—a skill worth practicing. It goes hand in hand with listening to ourselves and tuning into our own needs and emotions.

"Find gratitude.
It might seem counterintuitive,
but gratitude is a spiritual principle you
can practice even if you have a serious
chronic illness/condition. Wherever you
can and as often as you can, identify
things to be grateful for." [31]

My gratitude towards my family and friends runs deep, and feeling this way lifts my health to match every single day. The cirrhosis diagnosis and all that goes with it has changed me deeply. There is no turning back and I would not want to. This isn't a diet, a temporary fix, or a drudgingly tiring ordeal; it's become a huge blessing in disguise. If you're reading this right now because you are seeking something to get you through your day, know that you are not alone. Ever.

---

[31] [31]"Learning to Live Well with Chronic Illness/Conditions | Psychology Today," accessed March 18, 2023, https://www.psychologytoday.com/us/blog/some-assembly-required/201601/learning-live-well-chronic-illnessconditions.

Hope, Healing and Healthy Rewards

In my younger years, I had a beautiful horse. Her name was Lightning Bug and I purchased her from a livery string back in the early '80s. A livery string, as they call it in the horse world, is a place where one can rent a horse to ride on the trails. I had taken riding lessons as a very young girl and always dreamed of owning a horse of my own. I was a horse-nut through and through. As I grew healthier and closer to my goal weight, I began dreaming of getting back in the saddle again. This could be a new way to be more physical in life. I had been unable to ride for several years due to my knee injury and my weight. Stables required you to be under a certain weight to ride. Having owned a horse, I also understood the danger of falling off. Besides the fear of injury, the thought of getting back in the saddle with my bum leg concerned me. Would I have the strength to lift myself up on the horse and swing that leg over the saddle? Setting this personal goal for myself gave me a positive space to look toward. This was a passion I could rekindle if I kept my focus on health strong.

In the meantime, I had purchased myself a cute little blue bicycle. I named her "Little Blue" and I set to riding her while I waited for my body to be strong and lean enough to handle a horse again. When I first rode Little Blue, my legs trembled, and I had been sure my lungs were going to burst. We had camped in a spot with dirt and gravel roads in a higher altitude and it made pedaling a challenge. But I had done it, and I then had a new source of exercise to keep me interested. Walking had been wonderful, but it sure was fun to go fast! Variety was key, and it set my mind to dreaming, and I had thought to myself. "I think I'm ready. I can taste it, feel it even. I can smell the horse, leather, the barn. I can feel the rocking stride, hear the groan of the leather and the chomp of the bit. The wind is picking up my hair and fills my lungs, sending more healing blood throughout my body." I needed to find a stable to fulfill that dream.

I found the perfect place to realize my dream when our travels led us back to Texas in April of 2022. That prior April, we had been in the same location. It brought back the memories of my emerging health crisis when we set up camp once more. This was a prime example of full circle. I had set my sights to change on April 12, 2021, not knowing how life was going to play out. Then, in April 2022, I was over 100 pounds lighter, armed with test results announcing my successful healing, and all my new healthy habits were in place. The research, nutrition, exercise, and self-care had been, for the first time in my life, showing me what my new future held. It was very exciting to realize how much power I had, when I focused my energy in the right place. The hard work had been paying off.

I found a private stable which offered trail rides, and I reached out to the owner. After chatting with her I set up a one-on-one lesson, and a four-hour trail ride to follow a few days after. It was important to me to reacquaint myself with riding properly. I hadn't wished to injure my new, healthy body. The stable was a private one, and the horses on site were all meticulously cared for and quite well loved. The bonus here was these horses were all some of my favorite, bucket list breeds! I won't bore the non-horse people here, but trust me when I say, I was in heaven. I had taken my good camera with me, and arrived a little early to fulfill my love of photography. I was always thinking of having good photographs on hand for future art projects. It had become natural to me to combine interests. Hiking and photography gave me an excuse to get outside, while the photographs helped me to create art. So I set off taking photographs of the horses. Neil came with me, and listened to me chatter on, so excited to tell him what each horse breed was. He listened as I marveled at their beauty. He likes horses, don't get me wrong, but he isn't a horse nut. Sorry, honey.

I met the owner as I wandered, and she showed me the foals and allowed me to photograph them as well. We then chose a trusty steed for me. So up I went on Jewel, a stunning palomino Tennessee Walker. Trained in verbal and body commands, she responded to the slightest movement. A gentle squeeze of the leg, a lean forward or back, a click of the tongue brought immediate response. I learned to communicate with her during this lesson so we would be in tune. For me, it was love at first ride. We clicked.

Communicating with an animal is how we need to communicate with ourselves. Be alert, pay attention, send gentle yet firm instruction, and follow through. I felt nothing but joy and confidence being back in the saddle again. We had some laughs when communication failed and she responded in kind. You don't lean forward unless you mean it. She stops on a dime. Oops! I survived the lesson recharged and ready for my trail ride a few days later, which was off-the-chart wonderful. I will tell you that one of the unexpected hazards of losing so much weight led to an extremely sore bum the next morning. All my extra "floof" was gone. Good trade.

This was an example of what my big reward looked like. The beauty is I can do it again and again, and have done so as we travel across the country. Never will the experience be as sweet as that first time. I went home that very night and created a portrait in pastels of one of the fillies I met that day. I gifted the portrait to the owner of the stable in thanks for her hospitality. It was a gift to myself as well to be able to share that joy with another.

Rewards may come in the form of purchasing new clothes. Find a healthy restaurant for a meal with friends or invest time in a passion you have always dreamed of. Find a new path to walk, discover a new author. The possibilities are endless. Listen to your heart and make it happen. Your reward can be anything large or small. The biggest gift to myself was seeing my own value. I now care enough about myself to create a healthy body, heart, and mind and release what held me back. I allowed the best parts of myself the strength to fly (or ride) once more.

Shadows and Clouds

One reason I adore art so much is that to create something interesting requires an understanding of values. If I don't place enough emphasis on the shadowy part of the subject, the brightest portions would never pop. The painting would be flat and lifeless. In photography, depth and shadow unveil the most dramatic shots. In nature, a good thunderstorm at sunset over a mountain range, when the sun suddenly peeks over the edge, is magical! It takes the breath away. We can't see the depths of the darkness, but the light that shines above it is almost blinding once it reveals itself.

Life mimics art and nature in many ways. Those of us with liver disease all start out with well-defined darkness. I've talked to quite a few people from the newly diagnosed, all the way to seasoned veterans. Most of them are still trying to figure out new symptoms. They are struggling with frustrations during doctor and hospital visits, or can't find sound information on how to eat. There are those who have lost a spouse, sibling, parent, or child to this often-unfathomable condition. While the causes, symptoms, and reactions of our bodies can be like night and day, case by case, there are many common threads. The most common similarity is the initial fear. A fog rolls in, and they're still in there, trying to live their lives, but this shadow dims their vision, their drive, and their desire to thrive.

One of the things that helped me to lift that darkness was opening up about it. Not being embarrassed or afraid, but being vulnerable by laying it out there. Partly because it makes me examine what's happening, almost as a third-party observer. Instead of sitting in the muck and stewing, I look from above from an observer perspective and ask:

Susan R. Pryde

- What needs to be done?
- If she (myself) were my best friend, what would I want for her?
- What would I give to her?
- Would I let her sit there like that and suffer? Of course not!

Is it scary? Yeah, it is! It seems so much easier to hunker down and let someone take the reins. But who? If I wait for each appointment, each test result, and each opinion before I take action, I'm still miles behind in my recovery, aren't I? I'd rather read, study, learn, connect, and maybe, just maybe, learn something that puts me closer to the truth than slide further into the darkness. Sure, I'll slip. I might choose wrong, but at least I'm putting some groundwork down to have choices to examine.

I made a conscious choice to chuck damaging things out of my life, one by one: clean the house, and scrub away the dust; that's how I started. Once I felt that everything was gone that could hurt me, I was afraid to add things back. What if I choose wrong? I was afraid to eat anything at first, due to so many opinions out there. So, I had to turn off the chatter and look for facts. What is this sustenance here? Do I like it? Can it hurt me? Will it help heal me? If all the check marks are in place, I added them. If not, I will not add them back.

To all who are trying to figure out how to take that first step forward, it's out there, and you will find your way back to a better, brighter place. I cannot promise that everything will happen exactly the same, but it will be an improvement. Keep trying, keep learning, and make room for joy and laughter because that's healing, too.

Grieving

A common thread in chronic illness is grief. I grieved when I realized my liver was cirrhotic, at first because I thought my life was ending in short order. I grieved when I had to change my eating. While I became vigilant about every morsel I consumed, I saw everyone around me still enjoying foods I loved. I thought to myself, "Why did this happen to me? I wasn't perfect, but I certainly wasn't the worst eater! Was I? It's not fair! Why am I over here all bloated and unhealthy, and everyone else is still doing great?" It's too hard at first to look at the big picture, so I nit-picked and blamed myself for everything.

As I worked through all the physical, mental and emotional changes, and began to look within, getting past the grief was the one thing that continued to elude me. I would fall back into a sad "why me" space and wanted to curl up in a ball and be alone. It seemed so much easier to simply ignore it. Maybe it would resolve on its own? Nope, it doesn't work that way. I did not know how to express the fear of the severity of the illness itself, compared to how well I was feeling. How would I know that I could relax and go on with my life and let the fear go? I did not understand how to process the two sides of emotions I felt. I still did not know what the future held. I knew that I was feeling better than I had felt in years, but I didn't know if I could trust it yet.

I found an article in Psychology Today about ambiguous grief. An excerpt reads:

"...five reasons why illness ambiguity is psychologically difficult. First, ambiguity surrounding illness creates confusion. Am I sick or am I well? How will

symptoms appear today and how will they affect my goals, relationships and self-concept?" [32]

It was comforting to me to know that I was not alone with this grief. It was very real! How to deal with it from the same article reads:

"There are parts of myself that are forever gone; there are parts of myself that I am still discovering." "I am sick, and I am well." Practicing this skill involves slowing down our bodies and minds, attending to the present moment, and sitting with the "both/and" nature of reality." [33]

I experienced a continuous fluctuation of positive and negative emotions, going back and forth like a pendulum. Initially, the negative end of the spectrum would hold me captive for extended periods, making it challenging to regain a positive outlook. The fear of regression and jeopardizing my recovery, even the possibility of returning to the damaging effects of cirrhosis, would overwhelm me. But then, gradually, the pendulum would swing back to a place where I regained confidence in my own choices and allowed myself to acknowledge and celebrate even the smallest victories. Over time, my mindset began to stabilize more in the positive realm, providing me with the strength and resilience to keep progressing and flourishing.

---

[32] [32]"Chronic Illness and Ambiguous Loss | Psychology Today," accessed March 9, 2023, https://www.psychologytoday.com/us/blog/chronically-me/202103/chronic-illness-and-ambiguous-loss.
[33] [33]"Chronic Illness and Ambiguous Loss | Psychology Today."

*"You cannot go from
repressing/suppressing painful emotions
to being free from their grip without
specific approaches. You have to "feel to
heal" but if you were exposed to the full
force of your unpleasant emotions, it
would be intolerable."* [34]

By consciously addressing every aspect of my life that required a significant transformation, I unlocked the key to my healing journey. As I progressed, my grief began to subside. Removing the coping mechanisms I once relied upon, such as food and alcohol, allowed buried emotions to resurface, often overwhelming me. However, I understood that healing couldn't be rushed; it demanded time, patience, and unwavering persistence. For those who find themselves in a similar place, I hope my experience can offer some guidance. I've come to learn that transitioning from years of suppressing emotions to instant healing is an unrealistic expectation. When faced with a tangled rope of emotions before us, we cannot hastily sever or untie it all at once. Instead, we must slowly and methodically untangle it, allowing ourselves to heal from each segment as best we can. Attempting to flee from our emotions and life circumstances only delays the inevitable—they will eventually catch up to us, sometimes manifesting in physical ailments like cirrhosis.

Remember to be patient and compassionate with yourself. Recognize that not every moment of every day will place you in the winner's circle. It's okay to fully experience your emotions and learn from them. Embrace

---

[34] [34]"You Have to Feel to Heal: Emotional Awareness | Psychology Today," accessed March 9, 2023, https://www.psychologytoday.com/us/blog/anxiety-another-name-pain/202112/you-have-feel-heal-emotional-awareness.

days of solitude and quiet reflection and understand that shedding tears is a natural part of the healing process. Know that as you progress and acquire wisdom, those challenging days will diminish, making way for brighter, healthier, and more positive ones. When those moments arrive, allow the warmth and joy to permeate your being. Remember, you are deserving of it all.

Signs

Something began to change inside of me several months into this journey. I could not put my finger on it at first; I only knew that it felt "right". The day I truly awakened to this notion was in early October 2021. Our travels led us back to far western Arizona, for the second season since our nomadic life began. When we were there last, I was still living large (pun intended). Our visit then was going to be one of many tests of my new lifestyle. I had to firm up my resolve to keep going and learn to enjoy our time here in a different way.

Parked a few hundred yards from the Colorado River, there were lots of water activities. Among those were a riverside bar and restaurant, and a festive atmosphere. In the past, this would lead to fried bar food and riverside pina coladas. The task was to avoid fried foods and huge nacho plates, and pina coladas, while leaving the fun and adventure intact. I would eat before we walked to the beach or the tiki bar, take a long walk around the park or river before, and pack healthy snacks for the beach. At the tiki bar, I ordered sparkling water. If I had not already eaten, a nice salad with grilled chicken or shrimp was available and delicious. It still felt like a vacation but it felt different at first.

A few days in, I had the coolest experience. When I was young, I believed I was like Dr. Doolittle, and I could talk to the animals. I was sure I had a special kinship with them. For those younger than I, Dr. Doolittle was originally a series of children's books, and there have since been screen adaptations.[35] I am one who believes in signs, and what they might mean —what certain items or creatures we encounter might mean to us in a spiritual way. I had several experiences through the years where I felt that

---

[35] "Doctor Dolittle - Wikipedia," accessed March 9, 2023, https://en.wikipedia.org/wiki/Doctor_Dolittle.

tingle of importance. Moments the little hairs rose on my arms or a tingle up my spine that I couldn't quite explain.

Back to early October 2021. I had finished working for the day and gathered my water and my flip-flops to sit outside on the patio. I watched the people go by, the speed boats roaring down the river, and the ATVs kicking up dust. It always sounded like vacation here. Out of the corner of my eye, I saw the fluttering image of a little winged critter joyfully flittering toward me. It was weaving side to side, to and fro, making a sudden and calculated landing on my crossed knee. I gave a quick little intake of breath, both out of shock that she actually landed on me, and also because it tickled. Afraid to move or breathe, I sat regarding her for several moments. She stood still very light on my knee, only her little antennae quivering on occasion.

After about ten minutes passed, I called my husband over, and said "I think I have a new little friend. She's been sitting on me forever!" Neil was also surprised. We both expected our little fluttery friend to retreat now that I was talking and moving. Neil was peering down at her from above too, but nope! The little gal stood her ground. Neil went on doing whatever guys do around a campsite, and I was no longer paying attention to this creature anymore. After several more moments, she began to move. I thought "surely she will take flight now", and at this point I moved to see what she would do. I slowly crossed and uncrossed my leg. Still there! I moved my hands around and over her. Still there.

So I settled back into my original position and began to study her. It was here that she turned her wee face in my direction. Something in my heart clicked. It's that heaviness of a big emotion that hits out of the blue, sometimes. The shock of realization, or a feeling of joyful wonder, that is the only way I could describe it. My throat tightened, my eyes stung, and I was hyper focused on her.

I began to study her markings. I did not know what type of butterfly she was. Mostly black, with yellow-gold and white stripes, and little white dots, and she was not huge like some I have seen. Extended, her wings were perhaps the size of a half-dollar. I took photos of her as she rested and sent them to friends to help me identify her. We agreed that she was a bordered patch butterfly.

I googled the meaning of yellow butterflies, and general butterfly meaning. I strongly felt that her presence was a sign. I first looked up the meaning of an orange and black butterfly. *".. they represent transformation with honesty and integrity."* It went on to say that they *"... clear your confusion and overcome the struggles you're facing."* The last line caught me especially, that they *"...carry higher desires and thoughts and also shine light in dark situations."* Retrieved from Blogoguide.com.[36] This hit me square in the chest. My life had been turned upside down and I was then very much in a state of transformation and change. I had often felt deep confusion on how to face these changes. Would my friends and family accept the new me? Would I accept the new me? What and how much could I eat, what was the best way to keep my body moving? How on earth could I fit in this new world I was creating? Desperate to shine light on my situation, the darkness had been very deep. Physically, I was still very much healing as well, and I found myself often quite fatigued. There was still so much going on.

Curiosity struck me about the significance of a butterfly landing and lingering. So, I turned to Google once again while she rested on me to explore the spiritual meanings associated with butterflies. *"...a spiritual sign that represents you are in a season of transformation,*

---

[36] [36]"You Searched for Orange and Black Butterfly," *Dreams, Superstitions, Symbolic Meanings Guide* (blog), May 28, 2021, https://blogoguide.com/search/orange and black butterfly/.

growth, spiritual pursuits, and discovering your truth and inner wisdom. You are going through a deep internal change, even if you don't realize it.[37]

That was the day it dawned on me how profound my transformation was, and I needed to take my healing seriously. At that point, I began to talk with my little butterfly friend. I don't remember what I said, or even if I spoke out loud. She sat on me for one hour and faced me for the remainder of our visit. She would lift her forelegs to rub her little face or adjust her antennae. It felt like she was focused on me as much as I was on her. I thought of my mother-in-law, who loved butterflies so much, and I felt the strength of her presence. As if she knew how lost and afraid I was, she took this form to comfort me, to tell me that everything was going to be ok. I felt her telling me this all happened for a reason, and this change was good. I was going to make it through it if I pay attention and follow-through. My mother-in-law passed away in 2016 and she and I were very close. We often had late night deep conversations over the years. She was very much a mother to me, and a person I respected and emulated.

When my little friend finally took flight, I felt a brief sense of loss and sadness. I also felt a strong, excited vibration running through my body. She left me with a new, vibrant sense of resolve, deep in my soul that I was very much on the right track. Everything was going to be fine, if not better than fine.

---

[37] [37]Rose Putnam, "What Is The Spiritual Meaning Of a Butterfly Landing On You?," *Crystal Clear Intuition* (blog), accessed March 9, 2023, https://crystalclearintuition.com/butterfly-landing-on-you-spiritual/.

Part Three

HEAD

Susan R. Pryde

Knowledge is Power

Knowledge builds confidence. I found it easier to believe that I would heal as I began to understand how to eat healthy and practice self-care. I started to trust that I could make sound decisions about my health. So, while my health improved, so did my sense of self-worth and self-respect.

I now understand what healthy feels like. Living in a state of perpetual sluggishness and fatigue did not need to be the norm. In fact, it has become extremely rare now. Focusing on good health, rather than dwelling on having cirrhosis, was a game changer for me. This shift meant learning about my liver and focusing on ways to fix it, rather than on the fear of illness. Once I had shaken off the initial fear, and I began to turn my attention to what I could do next, my path became clearer. When I am faced with a difficult task, I still tend to stall for a bit, seeing only the whole mountain for a time. The difference is now I'm quicker to whittle it down into bite-sized chunks. This has affected my life in so many ways, for the better.

One piece of knowledge that escaped me in my research at first was that cirrhosis could be reversed. I googled this at least twenty times a day, hoping I'd find proof that I could do this. I found quite a few generalities, saying it was "sometimes" possible to reverse, or "rarely" reversed, but never anything profound. Then one day I found this video from the American Liver Foundation called "Ask the Experts: Acute and Sudden Liver Failure".[38] Yes, the title sounds ominous, but it is good news. Medical professionals are beginning to see more evidence that cirrhosis can be reversed in some cases (like yours truly). If you want or need a spark of hope, please watch this all the way through as they talk about evidence of the reversal of

_____

[38] *Ask the Experts: Acute and Sudden Liver Failure*, accessed March 9, 2023, https://www.youtube.com/watch?v=aleXOXHSO_s.

cirrhosis towards the end (around 22:15 if impatient). There is also valuable discussion about diet and other knowledge.

The Fatty Liver Foundation discusses the question of reversal of cirrhosis caused by NAFLD "*The message in this is that even with a cirrhosis diagnosis you are not helpless and there is a chance to improve your situation by learning how to stop the cycle of inflammation that is driven mostly by your diet. There are many ways to harm your liver but with our modern lifestyle fatty liver is one of the most common.*"[39]

Finally, something to hang my hat on, which gave me the hope I needed to keep going. Finding these nuggets of information helped me to realize that my efforts were worth the prize. I hope this book will also spark your desire to put your best efforts towards healing.

_____

[39] WAYNE ESKRIDGE | 573 40sc May 14 and 2018, "Can Cirrhosis Be Reversed? Of Course Not They Say, but What If," Fatty Liver Foundation, accessed May 16, 2023, https://www.fattyliverfoundation.org/reverse_cirrhosis.

Changes in Our Brains

I am reflecting on the changes that occur in the brain and cultivating the important ones to heal. I had to review all the dark thoughts, fears, obstacles, and imagined cliffs I envisioned in front of me. I saw them and felt that if I stepped off, I'd fall and never recover. The goal was to take those debilitating thoughts and address each one — to find the path around to a new way of thinking. The body cannot heal if our brain is battering our heart.

The biggest hurdles in my brain were the "what if's?" What if I would not heal? What if my days on earth were limited and there was nothing I could do about it? What if I really did not have the power to make changes and make them stick? What if upcoming scans and tests presented more health issues? What if my friends decide I'm too much work to hang with anymore? It was almost never-ending at first. My mindset was full of fear and anxiety.

I thought I may be getting medical PTSD, which apparently is a real thing! *"PTSD Symptoms: Re-experiencing is exactly what it sounds like: a mental re-living of the trauma. It can include intrusive thoughts, flashbacks and nightmares. For many people living with chronic illness, re-experiencing is particularly alive during interactions with doctors and hospitals. Driving by the hospital may cause panic; the prospect of both testing and treatment procedures creates tremendous anxiety."*[40] I struggled to sleep, especially before a test or appointment. I feared that every test result would deliver bad news every time. I did not fear the procedures themselves, but I greatly feared the future diagnoses. This was the case for

---

[40] [40]"What Does Emotional Medical Trauma Look Like? | Psychology Today," accessed March 18, 2023, https://www.psychologytoday.com/us/blog/afraid-the-doctor/202206/what-does-emotional-medical-trauma-look.

the better part of nine months. I knew I needed my sleep to heal but could not shut down my brain. I feared the worst outcome for every test or doctor's visit for a period of time.

The worst experience for me was the night before my EGD *(an upper endoscopy, also called an upper gastrointestinal endoscopy, is a procedure used to visually examine your upper digestive system).*[41] I had never had one before, and my support groups assured me it was a breeze, but I was still nervous. Neil and I had to leave early for that appointment, I had to be there by 6:30 a.m. and it was about a 45-minute drive. I could not eat or drink anything since a scope would go down my throat and I would be in twilight sleep. I woke up at 3 a.m. and I got up, and I tried to read poetry, check in on my support groups, anything to keep me occupied.

I found myself extremely dizzy that morning, lightheaded and shaky. My vision was blurry on and off. When Neil got up, I had to lean on him to get to the car. I felt like a very old, sick woman, and I was fearing they wouldn't be able to do the test, so it made things worse. We arrived at the hospital and checked in. All the while, I was clinging to Neil's arm for support, and trying to stop my head from spinning. Once we got into the pre-op room, my blood pressure was slightly low. Surprising, as that's the opposite of what you'd expect when you're scared, right? Otherwise, my vitals were ok, so they set me up to proceed. I did fine and had the BEST nap. I was a little wobbly afterward, as expected, but I was coming out of the anesthesia, after all. The nurses kept an eye on me a little longer to make sure my blood pressure was normal when I left. Going home was fine, but the whole event was a very stressful experience. The stressful part was in my head, not the procedure itself.

---

[41] "Upper Endoscopy - Mayo Clinic."

Susan R. Pryde

I leaned on my husband both physically and mentally those first six to nine months. I tried to remember that he was working hard to adjust to his new wife, who had been changing almost daily in front of his eyes. And he did so very well. I love that man!

My biggest challenge in the beginning was that I didn't know how to be in situations that used to be so normal. I had to do a thorough investigation before going out to a bar or restaurant, and at times the options were slim. No more bar food! So, I had to peruse the menu and approve the spot before the green light went on. I would look for a salad, and grilled options were a must. Many bars had only fried foods, and I chose to avoid those altogether. As long as I could get a salad with grilled shrimp or chicken in a small place like that, I was good to go. I also prepared ahead by packing my own food, eating before the event, or excusing myself to have a snack. I carried nuts and fruit, and my own stevia in my purse in case we were gone longer than expected.

I had no problem going out on the town and sitting with my friends while sipping sparkling water. A feeling of our togetherness was still intact, and I did still like the vibe. I did not find myself craving an alcoholic beverage or that awesome-looking appetizer. The most difficult piece of this was the knowledge, in my own head, that I was different now. I went back to the little girl in the corner of her kindergarten class who did not want to draw attention to herself. The worry in turn activated the spinning red lights over her head. "There she is!! The weirdo!"

Feeling different was such a big hurdle for me. Prior to diagnosis I used food for comfort and alcohol to hide my insecurities (hiding them only from myself, I now know). There were several things that helped me get through those awkward first months. Books were my friends! I found books that help readers overcome alcohol addiction or curtail their drinking. I also joined a "sober curious" support group. There are several such groups on social media, and I found a few that I connected with. One was a sober curious Noom group that I found on Facebook, and I found a few others that were formed from books that I had read, also on Facebook. Try a few on for size, I found some I could relate to, and you will too. These tools help people to navigate social situations where alcohol is very prevalent. The cool thing was the premise also helped me with my socialization in general. I related to these also with the food piece, because to me, it was one big, jumbled knot, and I needed to untie them as a bundle.

The first book I purchased back in the spring of 2021 was *This Naked Mind: Control Alcohol Find Freedom, Discover Happiness & Change Your Life* by Annie Grace. Annie Grace also offers an app called *The Alcohol Experiment*, both were a great tool for anyone curious about changing their relationship with alcohol. I did not use the app, but I could see how it would have been beneficial. I also found a support group on Facebook that is very active set up by the author. By the time I found her material, it was quite a while after I had been alcohol-free and well on my way with my diet. I found her tone to be engaging, non-judgmental and thought-provoking. I took my time reading this, as I was going back and forth at the time between that and researching food choices.

I got so much better in the first six months. Neil and I have now had several grand visits with dear friends and family and boy do I have good ones. They were gentle, understanding, put up with me and my quirks, and I love them for every moment. The very first visit of this kind was in September of 2021, a few months after my diagnosis. Living our nomadic life, we were lucky to land in places where loved ones chose to join us and vacation. There were often cabins in the campground we were staying in, or they would bring their own camper.

Susan R. Pryde

  While in Tucson that September, I was so excited to see everyone. Three couples were coming. I was stoked because I had not seen most of them in at least one year, when I was "pre-cirrhosis Sue" (well, I did not know I had it). For the most part, hanging out at each other's campsites, cooking meals, and going for hikes was perfect. My newly active, slimmer physique and mentality thrived on this. Then one day we headed to a sports bar to watch our favorite football team. It was the first time I had to navigate the food and alcohol situation, combined with all my fun friends.

  I built it up in my mind that this was going to be hard, so I made it come true. I set up in my mind that I would be the one person in the wrong jersey. The only one sipping ice water and eating a piece of lettuce, and all eyes and judgment would be on me. Let me clarify, no, my friends did not treat me that way, nor have they ever, it was all built up in my mind. I was cranky all day and grew increasingly overwhelmed and anxious. Returning home, while the rest of the group went to the pool, I begged off. I told them I had to prepare my meal for later (there were a bunch of veggies to cut, after all). Actually, I just wanted to sit and mope and feel sorry for myself. I'm pretty sure I cried. I could no longer be free and easy and not worry about hurting myself anymore. It didn't seem fair. I was very much like a child standing with my fists clenched refusing to have an enjoyable time. If they felt it, they did not judge me, I had to believe they could, and I did not want them to think I was judging THEM! Oh, how tangled it could be. I know now none of this is true, but it took some time to change.

  Later, I was able to shake this feeling off; my friends gave me space, then came and checked on me. They said they understood, but I needed to come out now and be with them. I did join them around the dinner table and enjoyed their company for the rest of the day. I told my buddies later that evening when asked how I was doing, "…you should live in my mind…it's always interesting in here."

I have learned to treat myself with a little grace and kindness — healing the body and the spirit alongside it. That was a challenge, too.

Finding Your Path Beyond the Fear

Fear can freeze you. I remember sitting in the corner on the floor of the classroom at age 5 crying because I was so shy. I didn't have the strength to join the class because I didn't want to be noticed, but guess what? The exact opposite happened.

My initial reaction as my diagnosis unfolded was fear. I was terrified, and yes, I did freeze briefly.

I began reading voraciously soon after my diagnosis, and quite a bit of that was figuring out how to find a positive and healthy path that must start from the brain. I needed to tap into that thick skull of mine. Here is an example of one I found and paraphrased below:

What are the 3 laws of attraction and what do they mean to me specifically?

1. Like Attracts Like: what it really means is that our thoughts attract our results. This is simply because what we think about and believe, we tend to do. Our actions then produce the results we have in life. If I wallow in negativity, that is what I will attract, so I need to believe that I can be healthy for this to occur.

2. Nature Abhors a Vacuum: it's like when you empty your junk drawer only to find it full of stuff a few weeks later. This is why Marie Kondo was correct when she said that *"tidying is life-changing"*[42] holds true. By creating space in our lives, we naturally attract new things. I had to eliminate the negative thoughts in my mind to make room for the positive ones. This also applies – in a HUGE way – to how I had to eliminate the food that was harming me and make way for new, healthy choices.

3. The Present is Always Perfect: the trick to activating the third Law of Attraction is to make your

---

[42] [42]"KonMari Method: Life-Changing Online Tidying Course," accessed March 9, 2023, https://learn.konmari.com/?campaign=ShfyNav.

current reality as perfect as possible. My husband Neil taught me to take action rather than simply whine about it years ago when I was unhappy at work and complained constantly. He said, "If you aren't going to do something about it, then I don't want to hear about it". I was hopping mad, but boy was he right! I'm not mad anymore, by the way. So today, that translates to, if I am going to sit in fear and complain about my situation, but never take the initiative to fix it, it surely won't get fixed.[43]

I had to find my way to the light at the end of the tunnel. At first, I could not see it. I didn't know what was wrong, I was afraid, and I felt very alone. Very dark. Each new medical test brought worse news, which would knock me back down. But a couple of things happened here that changed my world for the better.

First, I committed immediately to signing up for a weight loss program which I started on April 12, 2021, two days before my formal NAFLD diagnosis came in. I was so scared that I also dove in to begin learning what foods I should and should not eat in order to heal. Joining a weight loss program helped sustain me to get my calorie intake and mindset on the right path through to the next diagnosis of NASH in late April 2021, and then the final diagnosis of cirrhosis on June 15.

Second, I realized that to get through this I needed to fix where my head was at. It wasn't pretty in there, and I was that little 5-year-old in the corner of the classroom again. I had only Neil and Penny (our beautiful Boxer girl) to help lift me towards the light I was beginning to see, then our own children added to the mix of support — and that they did, indeed lift me up.

---

[43] Talane Miedaner, "3 Laws of Attraction: Start with the Present Is Always Perfect," *LifeCoach.Com* (blog), February 25, 2015, https://www.lifecoach.com/articles/laws-of-attraction/3-laws-attraction-the-present-is-always-perfect/.

Susan R. Pryde

I have always been a big animal lover. Penny has a light that shines so bright. Besides the benefit of having a walking partner, she brings that no questions asked love and comedy into our lives just when we need it the most. Neil and I fostered Penny back to health when she was taken from her life as a puppy mill mama (backyard breeder) in 2019 before we sold our home. Within weeks (our friends say they knew immediately we were goners), we knew we had to keep her. She's a beautiful blessing.

Third, I began to seek out reputable medical information on nutrition and my condition. Dr. Google scared me into action, but it was NOT a reliable source. I quickly found that so many sites on the internet that pop up in searches can be harmful. For example, many of the sites I landed on were for snake-oil type methods to "cleanse" the liver — promising quick healing if you bought their products, or just simply unscientific advice. Or worse, a random search led me to believe I had a limited number of days left on the planet, and let's face it, NOBODY knows when our day will come. So, I began reading about liver disease on Mayo Clinic, and Liver Foundation sites, and made lists for my new specialist to answer instead of guessing. I purchased a book called _Skinny Liver_[44] by Kristin Kirkpatrick, and it helped me to understand more about the liver, and what might be going on in my body, and how to begin taking the right steps. I also began journaling, and making the effort to do positive things for myself in the early morning hours, and I started a blog to get those feelings out and maybe find others who were in the same situation I found myself in. I needed to know there were others out there like me.

---

[44] "Skinny Liver: A Proven Program to Prevent and Reverse the New Silent Epidemic-Fatty Liver Disease: Kirkpatrick MS RD LD, Kristin, Hanouneh MD, Ibrahim: 9780738219165: Amazon.Com: Books," accessed March 9, 2023, https://www.amazon.com/Skinny-Liver-Program-Prevent-Epidemic/dp/0738219169.

Fourth, and certainly not the least important, I opened up and let my friends and family into my life. When I sat alone in the dark, it was hard to lift myself out of it. I had a wonderful little team that immensely helped me in the early days, and for them, I will be eternally grateful. I can never repay the encouragement and understanding I received. And then I grew braver and let everyone in. Having loving support in my corners was beyond measure. And they continued to provide it. I am thankful to so many for the roles they played in leading me out of that dark place, helping me see the beauty beyond. I had begun to live life more fully. I now know that I was completely healed, that I was capable, and that feeling was always evolving.

I had been reshaping my reality emotionally and physically since diagnosis. No, it was not easy, and I remain a work in progress. I had much to learn, but I was a willing student. My mind was open to new methods and paths, and I was determined to avoid anything that could hurt me further.

Susan R. Pryde

Letting Go

"The key to getting what you
want is letting go of what you've had." ~
Shawn Cassidy

During my morning reading while healing I came across a video of an interview between Shawn Cassidy and his brother, Patrick. The interview was interesting, and I loved the brotherly interaction. I had to admit, seeing a celebrity, who many years ago was the subject of girlhood daydreams, all grown up and a real human being was cool. He genuinely comes across as a great guy.

What struck me was when he said his initial success as a pop star at a young age made it difficult to move on. He struggled to know what to do with life after an overwhelmingly successful start at such a tender age. He realized it was to put it behind him and let it all go. Here was a man who seemed to have it all, yet was self-conscious about how different his life was, compared to his friends. His friends had gone to college, and he had not, and felt he would be perceived as "slow, "so he dove into reading books to catch up to them while he was raising his family. No matter the level of success we achieve, none of that matters if it doesn't align with who we know we need to be inside.

This concept of letting go resonated with me. There were so many things that I used to be that I thought I could no longer do or be anymore. While I loved my life and my friends, I was holding back and not doing so many things that were fulfilling to me. Growing up, I lacked confidence, which led me to be a people pleaser, often to my own detriment. I rarely uttered the word no, and I would seek out others' opinions before I dared to act on anything that interested me. This held me back both in my personal life and work, as I held back doing so many things that interested me, afraid that I would be judged or laughed at simply because I didn't want to appear different. I wanted to be invisible, someone who made no waives.

In essence, it is one hundred percent acceptable to live out the life that brings me joy. It was time to cultivate those interests, skills, and talents. I even avoided college because I thought my passions were not career-worthy. Why would I "waste money" on something I could never provide a return on that investment? Art and animals were my loves, and I couldn't see how I would ever make enough money in related fields. I thought I should do something "sensible." I decided for myself that pursuing my passions was a waste of money, so I opted to begin working and earning money instead. Thinking like this was not healthy, and I needed to rise above this deep-seated lack of self-esteem.

Prior to my cirrhosis diagnosis, the way I was eating was holding me back from walking or hiking in nature, riding horses, and doing activities that required a higher level of fitness. After diagnosis, the realization hit that I had to let go of who I was (the unhealthy me) rather than mourn the loss of (for example) eating fast food, or going to happy hour. I had to shift my focus quite profoundly or continue to live in a place of darkness, sadness, and "poor me." In reality, the things that I needed to change did not define the core of who I was. I was not the food I ate; I was not made better by wine. The changes I needed to make were quite literally going to make my life better, but I had to get to a place in my head where I realized this.

It was never in my nature to be down in the dumps, at least not for long. Oh yeah, I had bad days and sad days, but I was an upbeat person. I had a quirky sense of humor, I saw the joy in lots of little things, and I loved the company of my family and friends. Unfortunately, I had no idea how to crawl out of the space I landed in upon

Susan R. Pryde

my diagnosis. This was unchartered territory. My confidence was low. I had my feet planted not wanting to change, and I wallowed in sadness and anger, blaming myself for allowing my body to be so unhealthy. Looking back, nothing I gave up was important, not in any way at all! In fact, everything I gave up was holding me back from truly living.

Growing up and right up until diagnosis, I held back so much of who I was inside. I have found now that it is so powerful to take charge of the things that made me whole, and make room for them in my life. It is acceptable to write a book, create a painting, learn to crochet, make time for poetry and the beauty around me, and as I learn, I find myself doing so much more than I thought possible.

The Power of Letting Go by Melissa Kirk. It states *"But as we learned when we were kids, the other side of the coin of the fear of letting go is the jubilation when we spread our wings and fly. When we're pedaling furiously, and look back to realize our dad had let go of the bike minutes ago; when we're swimming like a fish underwater, suddenly realizing that we are, in fact, not drowning."*[45]

What Mr. Cassidy did to become the kind of man he needed to be is much like I did, without the credentials of the spotlight. Wait, I wasn't a successful pop star and a teen idol? Darn, what was I thinking? Letting go of old lifestyles and making room for new, healthier ones was a game changer for me. Letting go of comfort foods and alcohol left room to read, find fun videos like the one mentioned here, exercise, and broaden my horizons. As I began to eat better, I also felt better mentally. This new self-respect lifted my confidence. I was open to experiment with new things and fill my time with the big

---

[45] [45]"The Power of Letting Go | Psychology Today," accessed March 9, 2023, https://www.psychologytoday.com/us/blog/test-case/201203/the-power-letting-go.

---

things that made me tick. In turn, my outlook and confidence that I could heal my body grew stronger. I am letting go of the shy, self-conscious me, and letting the curious, passionate me take the lead. This version of me loves to fly.

Here[46] is info about the video I watched. If you loved Shawn, you may enjoy it. I did.

---

[46] *STUDIO TENN TALKS: SHAUN CASSIDY & PATRICK CASSIDY,* 2021, https://www.youtube.com/watch?v=yFy5PlGYrbE.

Susan R. Pryde

Building Groundwork for Change

There are many ways to view challenges that come before us. Our desire and focus to make change happen is the secret to overcoming obstacles. We have seen the past, but we cannot live there; we need to turn our eyes toward building a healthy future.

If you want something, you must silence the doubts, distractions, and fears. Halt that "drag your feet, why me, I don't wanna, it's too hard" rhetoric that we chant when something looms in front of us. Let's face it. We can always come up with a fine excuse. Not today — it's too cold, too hot, too rainy, and too windy. My mind is too cluttered today, I'm sad, I'm tired, I'm overwhelmed, I'm angry.

To change, we must take one step in another direction. I see where I wish to go, but I cannot find the road; where is the path to get there? It's all just too much. So don't look at every detail — pick one and conquer it. What can I change right now, what small thing? When you see it, grab it, make it happen, and make it stick, then pick another, and don't look back. Soon you will own the path, and you will love your journey.

Psychology Today discusses[47] the questions we should ask ourselves and provides tips on creating change. We must examine what we want, be willing to work and feel uncomfortable for a time and believe the change will benefit us.

It became important to create space for myself each day to learn who I am. I began with a sort of morning ritual of alone time. I rise before the sun. Early on after diagnosis, I was unable to sleep in because my thoughts

---

[47] "5 Essential Questions and 10 Tips to Create Positive Change | Psychology Today," accessed March 9, 2023, https://www.psychologytoday.com/us/blog/the-integrationist/201405/5-essential-questions-and-10-tips-create-positive-change.

were running rampant and I couldn't silence them. All the fears, questions, worries, and jumbled thoughts would arrive by 4 a.m. at the latest. It was either get up and start my day or lay there and become more agitated.

Keeping the lights dim, I prepare my morning coffee. While it brews, I weigh myself, take my morning medicines, and drink a large glass of water with half a freshly squeezed lime or lemon. I read my morning weight loss lessons, which are positive and full of nutritional advice. I choose what feels right that day to read. Sometimes it's passages from a book of poetry, or I will search the internet for information about liver disease, or something to promote a positive mindset. I open Facebook and catch up with what the members of my support group have shared.

I created my own health blog in September of 2021, followed by a private support group for deeper connections that are linked to the blog. I will often share to the blog and group quotes from poems, or tidbits that I have found in my internet search about liver health. On workdays, this means I have about 3 hours of "me" time before I'm on the clock. Using this time to learn, writing in my blog, or reading something soothing helps me create an outlet. This makes space for my interests, researching nutrition, and self-care. The blog itself helped me to get my emotions out, name them, and give them life. In turn, I both understand and stand behind my own needs in a much stronger way. This morning ritual gives me the space I need to continue to grow and build my own self-awareness and respect. This first habit of the day sets the tone for my day and helps me keep my focus.

I work full-time on weekdays from our rig, and prior to diagnosis I found myself very sedentary, sitting for hours on end in front of the computer. I now set a timer on my watch to get up at least once an hour, and to take a walk at lunch. The more I move, the better I feel, and getting outside mid-day with our Penny-girl (our Boxer) always helps to clear my mind and lift my spirit. Now that my meals are healthy, I no longer feel that afternoon sleepiness that so often plagued me in the past. I have a spring in my step as I walk, and I can go much further now. I do the same walk after work each day unless Neil and I take Miss Penny to explore the area. We love checking out state parks and nature preserves!

Another very important aspect is making way for healthy meals each week with food prep. Neil and I make sure that there is plenty of fresh produce on hand, pre-cooked lean proteins, and I make my own salad dressings and pre-roast mixed veggies. I go more into this in the health section, but it is also a very important part of healthy habits. It makes me feel prepared and strong. Early on as I was learning what to eat, I would stress over every meal. Now I am confident and certain that everything is at hand, eliminating my anxiety quite well.

I have been learning to become the observer in my own life. One thing that has helped me to rise above my illness was to detach myself emotionally from the issue at hand. To allow me to view it as an observer and make rational decisions on how to proceed in mending. A friend of mine, Tim Kaufman, shared something that struck me. He slam-dunked the key that unlocked the secret to my own personal journey from the darkness. I am grateful to Tim, who is a ray of sunshine each morning. I always look forward to his often deep and always positive take on life, despite his own battles.

"Rather than becoming the results of a hardship, we need to take control of our emotional interpretation of the situation. Thus allowing ourselves to grow spiritually. Allowing ourselves to make rational decisions without an emotional charge. Allowing ourselves to

flourish in the face of turmoil. Allowing
ourselves to be at peace and enjoying the
happiness in our journeys! Have a
wonderful day!" ~ Tim Kaufman

I am a walking testimony to this approach. I thank Tim for sharing, and for always bringing positive food for thought into the lives of others. Below is an excerpt of an article from *Psychology Today*, by Laura C. Meyer MS, titled "5 Mindful Steps for Self-Observation."

"We give our attention every day;
to everybody and everything. We are
listening, watching, observing: We watch
television, we observe other people, we
listen to others. We know how to give
attention, we are simply not used to
giving it to ourselves.
To give yourself attention is one
of the most loving, caring, interesting,
brave things you can do."[48]

We must be curious, self-advocate, love the process, and find our own unique answers without judgement.

Sleep is another important aspect, and creating a healthy sleep ritual is important. Our bodies need rest to recharge and heal. As I rise so early each day, I tend to turn out the lights by 9 pm every night. I disengage from social media about 30 minutes before lights out. Humorous videos or reading soothing things help me wind down. I will lay in bed with a low light on if I'm reading out of a physical book, or turn all lights out and read from my

---

[48] "5 Mindful Steps for Self-Observation | Psychology Today," accessed March 9, 2023, https://www.psychologytoday.com/us/blog/mindful-recovery/202109/5-mindful-steps-self-observation.

e-reader until I get sleepy. Often, I'm out in less than 15 minutes these days.

I am continuing to refine these healthy habits. Having to pick up and examine everything I was doing to make sure it belonged in my world has been cathartic. I have created a more joyous space, where I can stand tall in the knowledge that I'm on the right path and living to the best of my ability.

Forming a New Life and Simpler Changes

Change isn't always slow. I have changed more since my diagnosis than in any other time in my life. The depth of change relates to becoming a mother, wife, or grandmother, or the loss of a loved one. These are the ones that bring immediate and profound change. One personal change was going back to the hair Mother Nature made for me. I stopped dying it and let it become silvery. This change may seem smaller than the larger ones I've made, but I suspect personal changes like these mean quite a bit to more people than we care to admit. It is an emotional thing, our appearance. Maybe I'll keep my hair silvery, maybe I won't, but the real message is we do what is best for ourselves — that's the secret.

Sometimes adjusting the small things hit us the hardest. We put so much effort into those big changes, yet the small ones still smack us right between the eyes. When we decide to look them in the eye and take care of them, it's freeing. We must be gentle with ourselves and allow time to adjust. Health, self-respect, and patience are the keywords here.

Weight loss was a big change for me, mentally. Losing over 100 pounds took some getting used to. I was ready to feel better, and who doesn't want to buy cuter clothes? What I was not prepared for was how difficult it was to get used to the new, smaller me. For a long time, I saw myself in my mind as a 260-pound woman, and upon passing a mirror, felt a jab of shock run through me. Who was this woman? I did not recognize myself in photos. Between the hair and being ½ my former size, it was quite shocking. I had never seen myself this small before, nor felt so healthy. And now that I had embraced my silvery hair, I was mind-blown. Having my rituals in place so firmly has helped me to come to terms with this change and accept myself for who I am now. It is a blessing, not a curse.

Susan R. Pryde

Feeling like a teenager while looking like a mature woman took me awhile to wrap my head around. It is a privilege and a gift to be able to age. This very gift is what I have given myself by choosing to live life in a healthy way, rather than continue as I was. I am maintaining what I consider to be a healthy weight, not worrying too much about weight fluctuations of a pound or two. It is now all about health, and not a number on the scale. I did so by using the same tools I used to lose the weight, yet allowing greater portions of protein or healthy fats. I listen to my body now.

"...we talk of our bodies as separate from our minds, in dualistic terms, a concept rooted in the words of 17th-century French philosopher Descartes. This is one of the reasons why we have separated mental health from physical health, although in reality, they are both physical."[49]

I own who I am now. I love that my focus is on health of mind, body and spirit. The three combined keep my balance and focus firmly in a space to continue thriving. I am gaining confidence that the days of yo-yo dieting and quick fixes is over. I have tools in my pocket to keep each part healthy; whether it is my food choices, searching for new inspiration, or simply sitting still and feeling. I have choices now. At my fingertips is an amazingly rich library of resources and support.

The biggest change of all is the gratitude I feel for my liver. I needed to hear what she had to say. I don't know if I would be the woman I am today, strong and confident and healthy, if I did not have cirrhosis.

---

[49] [49]"Where Your Mind Meets Your Body | Psychology Today," accessed March 9, 2023, https://www.psychologytoday.com/us/blog/your-brain-on-body-dysmorphia/202211/where-your-mind-meets-your-body.

Part Four

HEALTH

Nutrition

Nutrition was my first focus. My major cause of cirrhosis was the way I ate. I was 260 pounds with a BMI of 42 in April 2021. A balanced diet is the best option for optimal health and healing, and many may think we know our surface "why". But for the most part, we all believe we are bulletproof until we are not. When I began searching how to properly eat, I found too many types of "diets" out there, so many that my head began to spin. I was afraid to eat anything and everything for a time. I finally found what I needed on the American Liver Foundation, Mayo Clinic, and Livestrong websites. I mentioned earlier the book *Skinny Liver* by Kristen Kirkpatrick, and I kept that within reach early on as well.

These sites helped me to calm my fears and approach my nutrition in a calm manner. I had a long way to go, and I needed to settle down and learn proper nutrition. As I mentioned before, I joined Noom and started logging my food and calories on April 12, 2021. I felt I needed the accountability that a structured program offers. It helped me to look at weight loss in smaller pieces, rather than the mountain looming in front of me. I aimed to consume approximately 1,200 calories a day.

After beginning our nomadic life in the fifth wheel in the fall of 2020, I lived like I was on vacation. Patty melts, onion rings, big breakfasts, happy hours. If it hung from a tree or grew out of the ground, it did not get consumed unless it was laden with butter in the pan, or a rousing layer of batter. We all know that one person who ate cheesy poofs, smoked like a chimney, drank every day with dinner, never exercised, and lived to 93 (proven by that photo at that birthday party blowing out candles amidst the wailing of smoke alarms). Yeah, that guy (or girl). That's going to be me! Uh, no.

Not to say I was unhealthy my entire life. I yo-yo dieted around different methods of getting slim. And let me emphasize the focus of getting slim in and of itself. I did not focus on true nutrition, and in some cases, I did not realize my focus was off. Back in the '80s, I tried a diet a famous person did, and boy did I get slim! I drank only shakes, and a cheat was nibbling sinfully on a smidge of iceberg lettuce with the fridge door open so I would be stealthily unseen. I followed a big commercial diet plan on and off for YEARS, counting other indicators instead of calories. I relied on fat-free or nutritionally empty snacks that were 100 calories or less to try to stave off the hunger. I did toss a few natural foods in for good measure here and there. I succeeded then, too! On getting slim, that is, to varying degrees each time. But each time my brain said, once I was "done" I could have this or that again. And the cycle would continue. In my head, I never figured out how to make it a life plan, nor find my forever way of eating. This was all my doing, not the diet plans themselves.

I developed hypothyroidism somewhere along the way. I probably confused the heck out of that little nugget. As I began to research, it made me wonder about the connection between my thyroid and liver disease. To paraphrase an article from Piantanida E et al., "The Interplay between Thyroid and Liver: Implications for Clinical Practice," Journal of Endocrinological Investigation 43, no. 7 (July 2020), [50] the thyroid and liver have a complex relationship that affects our health and wellbeing. The liver has important roles in activating and deactivating thyroid hormones, as well as transporting and breaking them down. On the other hand, thyroid hormones impact the activities of liver cells and its overall metabolism. When someone has an underactive thyroid

---

[50] [50]Piantanida E et al., "The Interplay between Thyroid and Liver: Implications for Clinical Practice," *Journal of Endocrinological Investigation* 43, no. 7 (July 2020), https://doi.org/10.1007/s40618-020-01208-6.

(hypothyroidism), it can cause abnormal levels of liver enzymes, which may be linked to problems with fat metabolism, fatty liver, or muscle weakness. Severe hypothyroidism can even mimic liver failure, showing symptoms like high ammonia levels and fluid buildup in the abdomen (ascites). On the other hand, hyperthyroidism (overactive thyroid) can also cause abnormalities in liver function tests due to factors like oxidative stress, blocked bile flow, or increased bone cell activity.

Yo-yo dieting is not good for the body. *"Just a few extra pounds can set off huge changes in your body. You get more inflammation, which normally helps you fight disease. And it can harm your heart and make you more resistant to insulin. Genes that can lead to an enlarged heart get switched on, too. Lose the weight, and you mostly erase these changes. But you don't totally reset, and the long-term health effects are unclear."*[51]

My last big weight gain prior to diagnosis was between 2018 and 2021. I developed sleep apnea and required a CPAP machine to save me from gasping for air. This was also when I reached the highest levels of cholesterol, triglycerides, and blood pressure in my adult life. As we also know now, my liver enzymes were up. High triglycerides are apparently a huge indicator that fat in your body is too high, and your liver is dumping it. *"Alterations in fatty acid and triglyceride metabolism lead to non-alcoholic fatty liver disease (NAFLD), which is a common consequence of overnutrition."* [52] In hindsight, I

---

[51] [51]"Your Body's Reaction To Yo-Yo Diets Explained," accessed March 9, 2023, https://www.webmd.com/diet/ss/slideshow-diet-yo-yo-diet-effect.

[52] [52]Michele Alves-Bezerra and David E. Cohen, "Triglyceride Metabolism in the Liver," *Comprehensive*

should have known something was up. If only I had been informed. I was out of breath from minimal exercise, exhausted, and so over myself.

Now I eat quite clean. Zero alcohol, zero soda pop, no refined sugar, limited sodium, no fast food, and nothing out of a box. I do eat lean proteins, tons of veggies, prepared many ways, fresh or frozen, and lots of fresh or frozen fruit. When purchasing pre-packaged fruits and vegetables, I buy unseasoned, with no sauces included. To bulk up meals I add raw nuts, mainly walnuts, because I love them but I change it up. I add flaxseed and chia seeds (or others) to recipes when fiber is lacking. I make my own dressings to keep sodium and unpronounceable things at bay. I love salmon for its omega 3. I will eat some cheese but not like before. I avoid those fake "is this really food?" slices and I go for the good stuff. I will eat high cocoa-content dark chocolate. I switched to unsweetened almond or oat milk in my coffee and use stevia, as my doctor approved that for my coffee.

I know that some may prefer to see a systematic presentation of the way I am eating now, so I will give you two general lists. The lists that follow are not complete, but they are some of my favorites. I don't eat things that I do not like. I experiment! I pay attention to my body when choosing new things. Being aware of our unique medical conditions while building a menu is important. Here as well is the American Liver Foundation's nutritional advice:

"If you're a liver patient, your diet is adjusted to meet your individual needs. Talk to your doctor about what's best for you. Still, here are some general food tips for a healthy or healthier liver:

Physiology 8, no. 1 (December 12, 2017): 1, https://doi.org/10.1002/cphy.c170012.

What to avoid: Don't eat foods high in fat, sugar and salt. Stay away from a lot of fried foods including fast food restaurant meals. Raw or undercooked shellfish such as oysters and clams are a definite no-no.

Talk to your doctor about alcohol and your liver health: Depending on the state of your liver, you should avoid alcohol. If you're allowed alcohol, limit it to no more than one drink a day if you're a woman and two drinks a day if you're a man.

Eat a balanced diet: Select foods from all food groups: Grains, fruits, vegetables, meat and beans, milk, and oil.

Eat food with fiber: Fiber helps your liver work at an optimal level. Fruits, vegetables, whole grain breads, rice and cereals can take care of your body's fiber needs.

Drink lots of water: It prevents dehydration and it helps your liver to function better."[53].

---

[53] [53]"Liver Disease Diets: Fatty Liver Diet and More," June 15, 2022, https://liverfoundation.org/health-and-wellness/healthy-lifestyle/liver-disease-diets/.

What Do I Eat ?

Foods I embrace

- Fruits: apples, oranges, berries, pears, peaches, plums, bananas, melons, pineapples
- Vegetables: broccoli, cauliflower, asparagus, tomatoes, peas, sweet potatoes, brussels sprouts
- Protein foods: eggs, dairy products, seafood, lean cuts of meat, and poultry
- Legumes: beans, lentils, chickpeas
- Nuts: walnuts, almonds, cashews, pistachios, macadamias, pecans
- Seeds: pumpkin seeds, flaxseed, chia seeds, hemp seeds
- Whole grains: quinoa, oats, brown rice, buckwheat, and sprouted bread
- Heart-healthy fats: olive oil, avocados, avocado oil, salmon, nuts, seeds
- Dark chocolate: over 85% or higher cocoa content

Beverages

- Water, coffee, tea

Herbs and spices

- Black pepper, turmeric, ginger, cinnamon, cumin, dill, parsley, thyme, GARLIC (lol)

Sugar substitutes (in moderation)

- Stevia, monk fruit, raw organic honey or maple syrup

Foods I avoid

- Sugar: cakes, pies, soda
- Artificial sweeteners: aspartame, saccharin, sucralose
- Highly processed foods: fast food, convenience meals, canned soups, packaged snacks
- Unhealthy fats: margarine, vegetable shortening, fried foods
- Salty snacks: chips, crackers, pretzels, microwave popcorn
- Processed meats: hot dogs, sausage, deli meats, bacon, beef jerky
- High sodium condiments: soy sauce, teriyaki sauce, steak sauce, spaghetti sauce
- Raw or undercooked foods: raw or undercooked meat, poultry, eggs, unpasteurized milk, fish, oysters, shellfish, or mussels
- Alcohol: wine, beer, spirits, cocktails

I do increase my caloric intake somewhat if I'm super active. It is important not to undereat. I consume the most nutritionally dense foods I can find that also help with inflammation, foods that build up the body to protect against further damage. I am constantly reading and seeking out new combinations to make meals interesting. I eat three meals a day with a variety of protein, fruits/veggies, and nuts/seeds in each, and I have one evening snack. I start each morning with a big glass of water with ½ of a fresh lime/lemon squeezed in before I consume another thing.

I am not generally hungry the way I'm eating. I'm very satisfied. I don't snack anymore, and I used to need a feed bag. The foods I consumed in the past were laden with empty calories that left my body undernourished. There is no nutritional value in refined sugars, unhealthy fats, and highly processed foods. By replacing processed foods with whole, nutritional food, filled with fiber, vitamins and healthy oils, I am now getting the fuel my body requires to function properly and feel satisfied. I envision myself healing from the inside out with every bite I take. With the shift in focus to fueling/healing my body, rather than losing weight, my body responded in all the right ways.

It's a balance that I am still working on. I continue to watch my calories, I am still experimenting with how my body reacts to quantities and types of foods. I am learning to eat more intuitively, paying attention to my body's signals, not just the number on the scale. I have found that eating the purest, least processed foods is quite satisfying. After cutting refined sugars out of my diet, my sweet tooth is minimal, and I can and do enjoy an occasional treat without worry. Please know when I say "occasional" treat I mean special occasions, or once or twice a month in moderation. I did not focus on getting slim; instead, I set my heart on achieving the healthiest version I can be. Being slim now is a bonus that affords me the ability to live longer, be active, ride those horses, and hike those trails.

I reached my weight goal in December of 2021 by following these methods. Food can be our medicine or our poison. I chose medicine, and you can too!

Susan R. Pryde

Healthy Fuel for Breakfast

Learning to tweak my favorite meals to be healthy and satisfying was of utmost importance. Finding a balance in foods that provided energy and substance became my number one goal. Making healthy weight loss a priority while learning nutritional balance was overwhelming, to say the least. Pre-diagnosis I did not understand what my body needed to function optimally, and often my goal was simply to lose weight. As I researched post-diagnosis, my new goal was to eat nutritionally sound for my body feeding it the energy required to heal and live fully. I needed to eat in a way that would sustain me for the long haul.

"All foods supply calories for energy, but not all calories are equal. Foods that give you energy provide more vitamins and minerals for the amount of calories they supply, so choose nutrient-dense options to fuel your daily needs Simple carbs like table sugar are broken down quickly and are a fast source of energy, but eating them in excess will lead to fat storage. For a more steady release of energy, choose complex carbs, which are found in whole grains such as wheat pasta and brown rice. Choose lean sources of protein like chicken breast or beans, and heart-healthy fats such as avocados and nuts."[54]

One example of a tweak is in one of my favorite breakfast options. Here is what I used to eat on healthy eating days, versus what I eat today. The same base meal improved. Estimated calories are for reference only.

_____

[54] [54]"How Does the Food We Eat Actually Give Us Energy?," LIVESTRONG.COM, accessed March 9, 2023, https://www.livestrong.com/article/444740-how-does-the-food-we-eat-actually-give-us-energy/.

Pre-cirrhosis breakfast:

- 113 gm low fat cottage cheese – 90 Cal
- 1 clementine orange – 45 Cal
- 1 medium banana – 105 Cal
- ½ serving (based on ¼ cup serving) store - bought granola – 60 Cal
  - Estimated total – 300 Cal

Post diagnosis with healthy changes in place

- 113 gm low fat cottage cheese – 90 Cal
- 1 clementine orange – 45 Cal
- 70 gm mixed berries – 32 Cal
- 14 gm raw walnut pieces – 90 Cal
- 1 tbsp ground flaxseed– 40 Cal
- 1 sprinkle each cinnamon, turmeric, and ginger spice – approx. 20 Cal
  - Estimated total – 317 Cal

What makes post-cirrhosis breakfast better than pre-cirrhosis breakfast you may wonder? The few calories added were well worth the switch. I found that my pre-cirrhosis breakfast did not satisfy my hunger for more than an hour or two. I could not live in a perpetual state of hunger; oh no, that would not do. I kept the cottage cheese because I love it and opted to tweak it elsewhere. I am not lactose intolerant, and as I had already eliminated all added salt, I felt comfortable eating it. Check labels on your favorite brands, cottage cheese can be high in sodium, and if that is an issue for you, be aware. A substitution of yogurt fits in here as well.

*"Long considered a health food,
especially if it is low-fat, cottage cheese
is a rich source of essential nutrients,
including calcium and protein. Because
your body digests cottage cheese slowly,*

it is prized by athletes, fitness buffs or anyone who wants to stay well-nourished throughout a long day. Naturally low in acid, cottage cheese might help with indigestion, but if you are lactose-intolerant or mixing it with meat products, it might cause heartburn."[55]

The clementine stayed, partly because I adore the taste combination of the creamy cottage cheese and the tart, sweet fruit. I wanted vitamin C and fiber. I switched the banana to berries both for the calories and the health benefits of berries. Yes, I still eat bananas, but I loved the fiber and antioxidant benefits in the berries. Also, I was seeking foods that would help with inflammation. *"Because of their rich antioxidant content, blackberries and blueberries have been called "anti-cancer" fruits that can also help protect against other chronic diseases like heart disease and arthritis."[56]*

I eliminated store-bought granola. Processed granola can be full of preservatives, sugars, and sodium so I replaced it with raw walnuts. *"High in fat and calories, walnuts might not be considered a weight loss wonder food. But think again. Their protein and fiber may help fight hunger pangs, their healthy fats may have positive effects on hormones that control appetite, and they may stimulate*

------

[55] [55]"Cottage Cheese and Digestion," LIVESTRONG.COM, accessed March 9, 2023, https://www.livestrong.com/article/502258-cottage-cheese-and-digestion/.

[56] [56]"Nutritional Value of Blackberries & Blueberries," LIVESTRONG.COM, accessed March 9, 2023, https://www.livestrong.com/article/527147-nutritional-value-of-blackberries-blueberries/.

areas of the brain that make food choices."[57] I have opted to make natural food choices wherever possible, and this was an easy choice. Walnuts added the crunch I desired, without food label confusion.

A nice addition was the ground flaxseed. *"The omega-3 fatty acids in flaxseed promote heart health and brain development. The fiber in flax can help smooth digestion, protect colon health and reduce cholesterol levels. Flaxseed is the richest source of lignans, phytochemicals that may play a role in preventing chronic diseases such as cancer, heart disease and osteoporosis."*[58] I buy flaxseed whole and grind it myself, storing whole seeds in a cool, dry place. I place the ground seeds in a small container for quick food preparation each morning. Keeping flaxseed like this helps to preserve it longer.

The addition of spices is for flavoring and the benefits of each. Cinnamon helps with inflammation, heart health, blood sugar levels, and brain health.[59] Ginger is excellent for thyroid function, inflammation and nausea. Turmeric is great for inflammation and liver health.[60] I

---

[57] [57]"The Fascinating Link Between Walnuts and Weight Loss," LIVESTRONG.COM, accessed March 9, 2023, https://www.livestrong.com/article/13559046-walnuts-could-hold-the-key-to-weight-loss/.

[58] [58]"The Dosage of Ground Flaxseed," LIVESTRONG.COM, accessed March 9, 2023, https://www.livestrong.com/article/456688-the-dosage-of-ground-flaxseed/.

[59] "https://www.livestrong.com/article/495786-is-a-teaspoon-of-ground-cinnamon-good-for-you/.[59]"Is a Teaspoon of Ground Cinnamon Good for You?," LIVESTRONG.COM, accessed March 9, 2023, https://www.livestrong.com/article/495786-is-a-teaspoon-of-ground-cinnamon-good-for-you/.

[60] [60]"Benefits of Turmeric Powder," LIVESTRONG.COM, accessed March 9, 2023,

would use all three spices for their anti-inflammatory use alone, as they helped reduce the size of my liver.

I have done my best to research all the best and tastiest foods to incorporate into my day. My post-cirrhosis breakfast has protein and fiber and is tasty enough to hold me until lunch. I no longer wish to gnaw on my pencil in starvation, which is exactly what happened before. Eating must be enjoyable and sustainable. If it doesn't taste good, it doesn't go in my belly. Altering my known favorites rather than choking down bland, tasteless food has been a lifesaver for me. This is by no means the only option out there. I could instead eat eggs, sautéed veggies, and a slice of sprouted bread as well, and I do! The important thing is to find the balance that keeps your mouth and tummy happy without adding stress to the liver.

---

https://www.livestrong.com/article/145900-benefits-of-turmeric-powder/.

You Can Always Eat a Salad

This is what people said to me a lot while I was struggling with eating out. "Oh honey, but have you seen MY salads? I think NOT!" My salads are a great meal, loaded with nutrition. One of my absolute favorites is my chicken fajita bowl.

Chicken fajita bowl ingredients (this is my serving)

- 4 oz boneless, skinless chicken breast
- 4 oz sliced onion and bell peppers
- ½ plum tomato – cut in small pieces
- 2 cup salad greens (I usually use a mixed blend, or spinach leaves — whatever I have on hand)
- 1 tsp of chia seeds
- 1 container of pre-packaged wholly guacamole (when I don't want to waste a ½ an avocado)
- 2Tbsp pico de gallo
- ½ plum or peach

I use the wholly guacamole cup, with the chia seeds stirred in as my salad dressing. Paired with the pico it is enough moisture and flavor for me. That eliminates the need to find one that isn't loaded with preservatives and sodium and sugar.

Neil prepares the chicken breast, sautéing together with the peppers and onions on his Blackstone griddle outside. A Blackstone is a large griddle with legs, made of cast iron and requires no oil to make a yummy stir fry. He does most of the cooking outdoors — he has quite the set-up. We marinate with Spanish paprika, garlic and cumin to taste, instead of using pre-packaged fajita mix. This helps us control what is in it, and we hold the salt.

Susan R. Pryde

This meal is about 350 calories of filling, nutritious goodness. My sweetie cooks the meat and veggies ahead and I portion it out and freeze some. He makes up about a week's worth of servings for me at a time. How can you go wrong with lean protein — check. Veggies —check. Power greens — check. Omega 3 — check. Seeds for bulk — check. Healthy fats – check. Sweet and juicy fruit – check. Spicy pico — check. Whole foods – check. And did I mention it's filling? I put these beauties in a bowl most people would use to serve the family out of and it's all mine.

Compare this well thought out meal with the average restaurant salad. Those lean toward bland, dry chicken, iceberg lettuce, a couple of grape tomatoes, and maybe a cucumber slice or two. Top it all off with a sugary, fat-laden processed salad dressing, usually totaling upwards of 700 calories and I'd rather eat at home. Salads don't have to be a boring meal. In fact, I don't call my meals salads, I call them power bowls. Resting on a bed of healthy greens is the only reason they resemble a typical salad.

Beets Me! Reducing Inflammation in the Body

Beets are a wonderful thing! This red, sweet beauty packs a powerful punch for my upwards climb to good health. Beets can be incredibly beneficial for ridding our bodies of inflammation and easing aches and pains. The betalains in beets make it a great anti-inflammatory option.

Betalains are natural substances found in certain vegetables, and beets are one of the few vegetables that contain them. There are two types of betalains in beets: betacyanins, which make red and purple beets colorful, and betaxanthins, found in golden beets. What makes betalains interesting is that they have the power to reduce inflammation and act as antioxidants in our bodies. In simpler terms, they can help fight harmful substances and protect our cells.

"According to a review published in Nutrients in 2015, betalains have strong anti-inflammatory and antioxidant potential and may prove beneficial in the treatment of such conditions as arthritis and cancer."[61].

I worked hard to find nutritional solutions for aches, pains, and to reduce inflammation. There have been studies that certain foods can help us. A whole food, balanced approach to nutrition and a healthy lifestyle combined is key here. So, I put beets on my grocery list and I love to roast them. They add a sweet and very RED

---

[61] [61]"Why Are Beets Good for You?," LIVESTRONG.COM, accessed March 9, 2023, https://www.livestrong.com/article/413049-why-are-beets-good-for-you/.

addition to my meals. They are also a good Halloween root if you want it to look like a horror show in the kitchen.

But let's not limit ourselves. There are plenty of other food options to enjoy. While beets can add color to our meals, it's crucial to have a variety of choices from the rainbow of fruits and vegetables. It's not sustainable to eat things we don't like in the long run, so it is important to be open and experiment with different foods. If beets aren't your favorite, don't worry or feel discouraged. There are numerous other delicious options available for you to explore.

According to a November 2020 study in the British Journal of Nutrition, dietary nutrition has a direct affect on overall inflammation as well as gut health in the body[62]. As I mentioned while discussing beets, it's best to focus on eating whole and plant-based foods. These foods include dark leafy greens like spinach and kale, which are packed with nutrients. Cruciferous vegetables like broccoli and Brussels sprouts are also great options. Berries, such as strawberries and blueberries, are not only delicious but also have anti-inflammatory properties. Including omega-3-rich fatty fish like salmon in your diet can be beneficial. Using olive oil as a primary cooking oil is a healthier choice. Opting for whole grains like brown rice and oatmeal instead of refined grains can help reduce inflammation. Spices like turmeric, cumin, cinnamon, basil, and parsley not only add flavor but also have anti-inflammatory effects. Adding ginger to your meals or having it as tea can be soothing for inflammation. If you have a sweet tooth, dark chocolate in moderation can also have anti-inflammatory benefits.

---

[62] Zheng J et al., "Dietary Inflammatory Potential in Relation to the Gut Microbiome: Results from a Cross-Sectional Study," *The British Journal of Nutrition* 124, no. 9 (November 14, 2020), https://doi.org/10.1017/S0007114520001853.

I have made every effort to incorporate these items into my daily meals. And for the flip side, certain foods have the potential to increase inflammation in certain people, depending on how their bodies react to them, like if they have a food intolerance. However, there are also foods that generally cause inflammation. These include sugar, refined carbohydrates like white bread, pasta, pastries, and processed foods with long ingredients lists. Refined cooking oils such as canola and vegetable oils should be avoided. It's best to be mindful of these food items to help manage inflammation in our bodies.

Eat well and be healthy!

The Right Carbs

Refined sugar is the big carbohydrate elephant in the room and it's not good for the liver. It causes inflammation that can lead to fibrosis and cirrhosis in some individuals. We find sugar on store shelves in almost everything in a box or bag. From bags of sugar for baking, to syrups, in boxed and processed foods, sweets, and in alcoholic beverages.

I needed to learn how to incorporate complex carbohydrates into my diet, guilt-free. In the past, I had tried to cut all carbs, but I realized that I had oversimplified the approach and had not understood the distinction between different types of carbohydrates. So, my goal became to add healthy carbohydrates to my diet while reducing the intake of simple (less healthy) carbohydrates. Nowadays, I make sure to have at least one serving of fruit and vegetables with every meal. I include some form of sprouted bread, seeds, or legumes with each meal as well.

An article about the difference in carbohydrates from Livestrong.com states:

"Foods made up of complex carbs are usually unprocessed or minimally processed, so they contain all or most of their nutrients and fiber — meaning that they're the closest to natural form…"and alternately "…You'll usually find simple carbs in highly processed carbs that have been stripped of most of their nutrients and fiber during the manufacturing process. Refined carbs include foods like white rice, white bread and white pasta…"[63]

Processed foods and foods stripped of their natural fibers are less filling, leave us wanting more, and make us

---

[63] [63]"Instead of Cutting Carbs, Choose The Right Ones With This Guide," LIVESTRONG.COM, accessed March 9, 2023, https://www.livestrong.com/article/35816-list-good-bad-carbs/.

sluggish. Fruits and vegetables, in their natural form, are full of fiber, vitamins, and nutrients that our bodies need to function.

We need to be aware of our individual dietary needs and conditions and how foods affect us. Be aware of the spikes in blood sugar they can cause in someone with diabetes or insulin resistance. According to an article in Harvard Health, *"Picking good sources of carbs can help you control your blood sugar and your weight. Eating healthier carbohydrates may help prevent a host of chronic conditions, especially diabetes, but it is also associated with a lower risk of heart disease and certain cancers."* [64]

Knowing the glycemic index in the foods we eat can help us make the best choices for our bodies. I found a handy tool here to look it up:[65] The glycemic index ranks food from 1-100 based on how quickly they are digested and get into your bloodstream. The higher the number for the food, the quicker it raises your blood glucose levels.

Go ahead and try out this glycemic index tool. I would suggest plugging in your favorite items to help you make informed choices. For example, if you are craving fruit, should you choose an apple, with a glycemic index (GI) of 28, or do you go for watermelon, with a GI of 72? In this instance, the apple is your winner. The same applies to vegetables, would you choose the carrots at 16 GI, or mashed potatoes at 68 GI? Grains have a winner in barley, sliding in at only 21 GI, while white rice is 92 GI. [66]

---

[64] [64]"A Good Guide to Good Carbs: The Glycemic Index - Harvard Health," accessed March 9, 2023, https://www.health.harvard.edu/healthbeat/a-good-guide-to-good-carbs-the-glycemic-index.

[65] [65]"Glycemic Index – Glycemic Index Research and GI News," accessed March 9, 2023, https://glycemicindex.com/.

[66] Fiona S. Atkinson, Kaye Foster-Powell, and Jennie C. Brand-Miller, "International Tables of Glycemic Index and Glycemic Load

Susan R. Pryde

The importance of choosing the right carbohydrates for our health is key here. Refined sugar is harmful to the liver, causing inflammation that can lead to fibrosis and cirrhosis. Processed foods and those lacking natural fibers leave us unsatisfied and sluggish, while fruits and vegetables in their natural form provide essential fiber, vitamins, and nutrients. Understanding the distinction between complex and simple carbohydrates is key. Incorporating healthy carbohydrates while reducing the intake of less healthy ones is the goal.

Awareness of individual dietary needs and conditions, such as blood sugar spikes in diabetes or insulin resistance, is crucial. Making informed choices based on the glycemic index can help manage blood sugar levels. Achieving balance in our diet is essential, particularly for individuals with liver disease, as it allows for better control of blood sugar levels and informed decisions about food choices and quantities.

Values: 2008," *Diabetes Care* 31, no. 12 (December 2008): 2281, https://doi.org/10.2337/dc08-1239.

Over-The-Counter Medications and Supplements

Medications and supplements pass through the liver, and caution should be the first rule of thumb. Review all with a medical professional before taking. This is exactly how I approached both, so I am sharing direct quotes right off the bat on this subject.

An excerpt from the Mayo Clinic on over-the-counter medications states:

> *"Are pain medications safe to take with liver disease?*
>
> *Well, some pain medications are safe to take in certain doses, and some are not. For instance, nonsteroidal, anti-inflammatory drugs such as ibuprofen and naproxen should be avoided in patients with cirrhosis, because when the liver is scarred, there's a greater chance of hurting the kidneys with these types of medications. Narcotics such as oxycodone are not a good idea either as they can be quite problematic with certain complications of cirrhosis. Acetaminophen, on the other hand, is safe to take, but at smaller doses. For pain relief in cirrhosis, we recommend taking acetaminophen up to two grams a day. So that's four extra strength tablets within a 24-hour period."*[67]

The same article addresses supplements:

---

[67] [67]"Cirrhosis FAQs," Mayo Clinic, accessed March 9, 2023, https://www.mayoclinic.org/diseases-conditions/cirrhosis/multimedia/vid-20532300.

Susan R. Pryde

*"Will taking supplements help
my cirrhosis?*
*Although certain herbal
supplements such as milk thistle have
been tried in liver disease, there's no
evidence to suggest that herbal
supplements or any other alternative
therapies can effectively treat cirrhosis.
However, there is a chance of herbal
supplements causing harm to the liver,
sometimes to the point of liver failure
requiring a liver transplant. So we
recommend avoiding any and all herbal
supplements".* [68]

The subject of supplements and alternative
treatments are especially important, as there are so many
products posing as supplements, cleanses, and cures.
When I learned about my struggling liver, one of the first
things I researched was supplements. In the support
groups I was in, many people suggested taking various
things and doing "cleanses." I was tempted to follow their
advice without consulting my specialist, driven by my
desperation to improve my condition. However, it didn't
occur to me at first that adding more substances to my
already struggling liver to process might not be a wise or
safe idea before allowing it to focus on healing itself.

I like to say before changing my diet to whole,
clean foods, assuming any one thing would have "fixed"
me would be akin to tossing a deck chair off the Titanic to
stop it from sinking. No magic for that. As it turns out,
none of those things were approved by my doctor, and
thank goodness I didn't have a package of lord-knows-
what arrive on my doorstep via Amazon before I knew this.
I could have done far more harm than good.

------

[68] [68]"Cirrhosis FAQs."

While some things may be beneficial, always talk to your doctor first. You never know the reaction your body may have, what might interfere with other medication, or cause severe damage. Sometimes it is the quality of the supplements or the fillers they use. I focused on getting those nutrients right from the horse's mouth, i.e., the food it came from.

The liver and kidneys and gastrointestinal tract are designed to cleanse our bodies naturally, and currently there is no alternative medicine proven to treat liver disease. [69] *"There's little evidence that dietary cleanses do any of the things they promise. The fact is you don't need to purchase a product to cleanse your body. Your liver, kidneys and gastrointestinal tract do a good job of detoxing it every day. If you're looking to rejuvenate your body, focus on eating more whole foods, drinking water and removing highly processed foods from your diet."*[70]

Be cautious about what you put in your body. Keep it clean out there, kids. Do not purchase anything without a call to your specialist first.

---

[69] Mayo Clinic Staff Print, "Liver Problems - Alternative Medicine," Mayo Clinic, accessed May 20, 2023, https://www.mayoclinic.org/diseases-conditions/liver-problems/diagnosis-treatment/alternative-medicine/scc-20374505.

[70] Cynthia Weiss, "Mayo Clinic Q and A: 10 Nutrition Myths Debunked," Mayo Clinic News Network, July 31, 2022, https://newsnetwork.mayoclinic.org/discussion/mayo-clinic-q-and-a-10-nutrition-myths-debunked/.

Susan R. Pryde

Hypothyroidism, Metabolic Syndrome, and Liver Disease

I found out I had an underactive thyroid in 2006. A prescription of Levothyroxine was in order. Levothyroxine is a medication that is prescribed for three main purposes: to treat hypothyroidism (when the thyroid gland doesn't produce enough hormone), to reduce the size of enlarged thyroid glands (known as goiters), and to treat thyroid cancer.[71] I admit that at the time I thought hypothyroidism was the sole reason that I was struggling with my weight. I imagined that this magical medicine would put me at my perfect weight, requiring no effort on my part. It did not occur to me that I should change something I was doing. I accepted the medications as the only thing that could help me, and as the years went on, that dosage kept going up. Until now, post cirrhosis diagnosis.

Throughout 2021, as I made changes to my diet following diagnosis, I not only experienced weight loss but also noticed an improvement in my thyroid. To monitor this progress, I regularly consulted my primary care physician and underwent thyroid level tests every three to six months. As my liver health improved, so did my thyroid function, leading to a reduction in my Levothyroxine medication as per the doctor's guidance. I continue to monitor my thyroid function through regular lab tests and faithfully adhere to my prescribed medication regimen.

Researchers have discovered a connection between an underactive thyroid (hypothyroidism) and a condition called non-alcoholic fatty liver disease (NAFLD). To paraphrase a recent article it seems that thyroid

---

[71] 71"Levothyroxine (Oral Route) Description and Brand Names - Mayo Clinic," accessed March 9, 2023, https://www.mayoclinic.org/drugs-supplements/levothyroxine-oral-route/description/drg-20072133.

hormone imbalances can contribute to chronic liver diseases, including NAFLD, fatty liver disease caused by alcohol, and liver cancer. When the signaling of thyroid hormones in liver cells is disrupted, it can lead to reduced breakdown of fats in the liver and the accumulation of excess fat in the liver cells. [72]

I want to shed some light on another condition known as metabolic syndrome, as studies show a correlation between it and hypothyroidism. *"There is significant association between subclinical hypothyroidism and metabolic syndrome. It highlights the importance of thyroid function tests in patients with metabolic syndrome."*[73] Before my cirrhosis diagnosis, I had never heard of it. *"Metabolic syndrome is a cluster of conditions that occur together, increasing your risk of heart disease, stroke and type 2 diabetes. These conditions include increased blood pressure, high blood sugar, excess body fat around the waist, and abnormal cholesterol or triglyceride levels."*[74] Metabolic syndrome is also a serious red flag for NAFLD and liver disease. It is also associated with diabetes, insulin resistance, high blood pressure, sleep apnea, high cholesterol, stroke, and high triglycerides. When I look back to when I was first diagnosed with hypothyroidism, I can now see the path that led me to metabolic syndrome, and liver disease.

With a healthy diet and exercise, you may be able to reverse metabolic syndrome. The more I read, the more I see connections. There were so many health problems that in the past I saw as single events. This article struck a

---

[72] Viktoriya Bikeyeva et al., "Nonalcoholic Fatty Liver Disease and Hypothyroidism: What You Need to Know," *Cureus* 14, no. 8 (August 2022), https://doi.org/10.7759/cureus.28052.

[73] Sunil Kumar Kota et al., "Hypothyroidism in Metabolic Syndrome," *Indian Journal of Endocrinology and Metabolism* 16, no. Suppl 2 (December 2012): S332, https://doi.org/10.4103/2230-8210.104079.

[74] {Citation}

chord. *"What's likely happening is that in some people who are overweight or obese, the body starts to rewire itself metabolically, which ultimately leads to a state of insulin resistance,"* he says. *"That insulin resistance can lead to inflammation of the coronary arteries and an abnormal cholesterol profile,"* slowly leading to diabetes and coronary heart disease*[75]*

If my cholesterol was high, for example, I wanted to treat "that." If my blood pressure was high, then let's treat "that." It didn't occur to me that all these things were wonky as a team. By not addressing the underlying issues, I was putting flimsy stoppers in the cracks, while the ship continued to take on water. Getting to the bottom of what our bodies need to be healthy aids in filling the cracks. We have the power to get our balance back. With effort and focus, and treating the underlying cause, health can improve.

---

[75] [75]"What Is Metabolic Syndrome, Exactly?," LIVESTRONG.COM, accessed March 9, 2023, https://www.livestrong.com/article/13723809-metabolic-syndrome/.

Mysteries, Conundrums and Hypotension

Most of us have heard of hypertension, the dreaded high blood pressure. I had it, or rather, I was creeping up on it, before diagnosis. One thing I did not expect was for the opposite to occur.

In the summer and fall of 2021 while adjusting my lifestyle I noted bouts of lower blood pressure. I was having dizzy spells, so I had asked my primary care physician what might be happening. He advised me to buy a portable blood pressure monitor and I began keeping a record. He had also reminded me to make sure I was well hydrated. I recall feeling a little confused because I had been very conscious of my fluid intake and drank about 64 oz. of water every day. By that point, I was feeling confident in my nutritional status, so that was not to blame.

We were visiting our daughter and her family for the holidays. One afternoon in early January of 2022 I had a COVID-19 booster along with a flu shot. The next morning, I woke with muscle aches, a sore throat, and napped all day. I was out of it. I wrote this off as a reaction to one or both of the vaccines. I would feel better the next day. The next morning I awoke at 4 am. As I opened the bathroom door it was as if someone hit a light switch in my brain to the OFF position. I went down like a sack of potatoes and I came to lying flat on my back. I recall wondering why my daughter's dogs were barking in my room (I had no idea where I was). Disoriented, I sat up and saw my daughter coming toward me in the dark. I announced to her that I had a little problem and I'd fallen. She told me later I was talking in whispers, like a small child. She and my son-in-law got me up to the couch and

Susan R. Pryde

took my blood pressure. It was 83/45. This is low. Normal blood pressure[76] is 120/80.

I ended up in the ER where they monitored my heart and checked for deficiencies in my blood and fluids. They found nothing, no evidence of heart trouble, dehydration, or nutritional deficiencies. My sodium and phosphates were fine as well, so they decided I had a seizure and sent me on my way. I had mentioned to them during the examination I had epilepsy yet had not had a seizure since 2008. Looking back, it's possible that he made this assumption due to a lack of other reasons.

My neurologist and the primary doctor did not agree with this diagnosis. I called them both and we discussed all that happened. Because my liver is so important right now, I also informed Dr. Swendsen. It appears either I am an anomaly, or I have done so well that I don't need to be so strict on my sodium intake as I have been. Watching sodium intake is important with cirrhosis - like heart disease - due to the potential for hypertension. Liver disease presents as portal hypertension.

All three of my doctors and I have agreed to approach this new conundrum as if it was some sort of syncope which *"...causes your heart rate and blood pressure to drop suddenly. That leads to reduced blood flow to your brain, causing you to briefly lose consciousness."*[77] I had been ill from the dual vaccines all day Sunday and did not eat or drink much. Combined with

___

[76] "Blood Pressure Chart: What Your Reading Means," Mayo Clinic, accessed June 29, 2023, https://www.mayoclinic.org/diseases-conditions/high-blood-pressure/in-depth/blood-pressure/art-20050982.

[77] "Vasovagal Syncope - Diagnosis and Treatment - Mayo Clinic," accessed March 9, 2023, https://www.mayoclinic.org/diseases-conditions/vasovagal-syncope/diagnosis-treatment/drc-20350531.

my already minimal sodium intake, this made my blood pressure unstable.

I was prescribed salt tablets and advised to take my blood pressure each morning. I had to take it once while lying down, then again upon standing to see the difference. I kept a record of the results and shared them after about a week's time. My blood pressure would be normal while lying down, but the moment I stood, it was much lower, and I was dizzy as I stood up. After a few weeks on salt tablets, this began to lessen and the spells became rare. I went off the tablets after about two months. Although I still do not sprinkle salt on my food while eating, I will add small sums when cooking, and my blood pressure has been stable.

There are a few sodium-related issues that can occur with both weight loss and liver problems. One of them is hyponatremia, which occurs when too much fluid builds up in the body, diluting our sodium levels[78]. Another issue is called salt shock or vasovagal syncope, which is a fancy term for fainting. To test for syncope, doctors can check our blood pressure while lying down and then immediately upon standing. If there is a drop in blood pressure, it's a sign of syncope. They can also use a tilting table in the office to monitor blood pressure while changing the angle of the table. [79] When we lose weight rapidly or exercise excessively while not consuming enough calories, we may experience light-headedness

---

[78] [78]"Hyponatremia - Symptoms and Causes," Mayo Clinic, accessed March 9, 2023, https://www.mayoclinic.org/diseases-conditions/hyponatremia/symptoms-causes/syc-20373711.

[79] [79]"Vasovagal Syncope - Diagnosis and Treatment - Mayo Clinic."

nausea, or dizziness. This can happen because our metabolism produces too much thyroid hormone.[80]

Before I began my journey back to health I had quite the lower extremity water retention as well as in my hands. As with everything else, I wrote this off as being obese. Not true. Research has found that consuming excessive sodium can cause various harmful effects on the liver. These effects include distorted cell shapes, increased cell death, and reduced cell growth, all of which can contribute to liver fibrosis.[81]

Moments like these were reminders to me to continue watching my health and working to maintain a balance. Putting all focus on one area could lead to serious neglect in other areas. This was another example of self-advocacy and self-care; we must pay attention to our bodies and the signals they send.

---

[80] [80]"Dizziness & Nausea When Losing Weight Too Fast," LIVESTRONG.COM, accessed March 9, 2023, https://www.livestrong.com/article/425420-dizziness-nausea-losing-weight-fast/.

[81] [81]"High-Salt Diet May Harm Liver," February 25, 2016, https://www.medicalnewstoday.com/articles/307028.

Navigating Social Events

One year into my healing, we attended the wedding of one of our bonus daughters. She is the daughter of our best friends, and we love her like our own. It was a wonderful weekend affair, and friends turned family converged from all over. As you can imagine, figuring out how to eat and hydrate was top on my list. I was looking forward to living in the moment and catching up with loved ones. Being on the road, we haven't seen each other in some time.

Gone was the easy breezy go-with-the-flow days of pizza, pancakes, and wine. Every meal can bring stress when that stocked kitchen is nowhere in sight. We didn't have our fifth wheel on this trip, so my rolling kitchen was far away. With a diet mapped down to the last lettuce leaf, losing that comfort can make things a bit sideways. Staying with friends or a hotel meant a little extra forethought to stay on track. This was a test in learning to swerve with grace and not make these moments into a crazed scramble to stay focused. Like a child whose parents have removed her training wheels, off I was on a wobbly course.

Since we were going to be in a hotel for several days, preparation was key. I checked to make sure they would have a refrigerator in our room, and made a list of foods to help get me through. Having raw mixed nuts and plenty of fruit and veggies on hand helped to get me out of any jams where nothing healthy was available. Luckily the hotel served some things I could work with for breakfast — thank goodness for scrambled eggs and fruit. I googled nearby restaurants in case a meal on the town came up. Eating at restaurants can work if there is some sort of lean protein, vegetables or fruit, or a salad on the menu. I will choose the salad with the most vegetables and ask them to hold the bacon and cheese or candied fruit. If they have healthy entrees, I will ask for steamed vegetables and the leanest cut of beef. I take a box home most times, as portions are outrageous. I will ask for some sort of vinaigrette dressing and always on the side if it is a salad. Oh, and keep the water coming, waitress! The night we arrived there was a pizza party and I decided to order my own salad from a local restaurant. No big deal!

On the day of the wedding, I kept it light for breakfast and lunch with the hotel options and my room stash (remember those fruits, veggies and nuts I brought?). Once we arrived at the wedding I selected the healthiest options. The bride and groom had chosen local BBQ for dinner, which was amazing! I loaded my plate with veggies, and the leaner cuts of chicken and meat and avoided the sauce. It was delicious.

This was the first big event after being diagnosed with cirrhosis. Considering the changes made, I would be remiss not to address alcohol. When had I last attended a wedding or big function sans alcohol? Most likely in the baby-bouncing years. So it had been a while. Exposing myself to smaller gatherings through the months helped prepare me to handle this. I struggled with being an "outsider" in my mind relating to food and drink along the way with varying degrees of inner turmoil. Big parties and bashes test my limits, and I've bailed early on several occasions, using whatever escape tactics I could muster. As the group gets rowdier, the more I felt different, and the important thing is to know it's ok to leave when it's rough.

I read a few books that helped me to come to terms with my changes. I found a few references to being sober-curious early on, which led me to a book called *This Naked Mind: Control Alcohol, Find Freedom, Discover Happiness & Change Your Life* by Annie Grace.[82] I had read this early on and it helped me to begin to break from the feeling that I needed a glass of anything as a path to joy. I

_____

[82] [82]"Annie Grace," This Naked Mind, accessed March 9, 2023, https://thisnakedmind.com/.

also read a second book, titled *The Unexpected Joy of Being Sober*, by Catherine Grey.[83] I was learning to find my voice free of the social lubricant of alcohol. Both books provided me with the necessary tools to confront the issue of alcohol, while diet, exercise, knowledge, and self-care constituted the other important aspects. For many years, casual drinking had been a regular part of various occasions. And while it could continue to be for others, for me it no longer worked. The books were a valuable resource for me. They helped me gather my strength and learn what alcohol was doing to my brain and my body.

So this time, as soon as the dance floor opened up I said to myself "you don't need any liquid courage, you're dancing tonight!" And you know what? That's exactly what I did. I ripped that band aid off and danced all night long. The bride was gorgeous, it was a beautiful wedding and I had a blast. I felt young and alive, and so completely present. Upon waking the next day free of guilt or headache added another notch of strength in my belt. This weekend helped me to learn to navigate the dips and turns that are always in our path. Placing myself in difficult situations helps me gain strength and prepare for the next. Now one evening out is easy! In the beginning the thought of facing a few hours outside of my safe bubble at home made me panic. I was going to be just fine.

---

[83] [83]"Unexpected Joy – Just Another WordPress Site," accessed March 9, 2023, https://unexpectedjoy.co.uk/.

Susan R. Pryde

Q&A and Longevity

Since I reversed my cirrhosis of the liver, questions have come from friends and family. I will share some of my thoughts and my responses.

Your liver is completely healed, can you eat again?

I chuckle at this one. I sense that some may assume that eating must be horrible now, bland, and boring. This is far from the truth. I am 100% satisfied and believe in the changes made to my nutritional health, and my body and palate are very happy. I did not stop eating at all. I leave foods with zero nutritional value on the grocery store shelf, and there they will remain. My body needed me to discover the key to its optimal performance, and I am better than ever before.

To maintain this new, healthy body, I journaled my food and calorie intake for quite a while. After a while, I began to eat intuitively. I listen to my body's' signals and put the fork down when I am full. I have become pretty good at visualizing portions, and I keep my food scale handy for new items. Except for research in spices and food preparation for new recipes, there will be no change here. I have learned to trust and respect my own opinion and judgement. The work on my mental game has helped me much in this area.

Hey, you can drink on occasion again, right? Or drink skinny drinks?

Putting alcohol back into my life will not improve my health. I am healed, yes, but I wish to maintain a cleaner way of living to remain at my best. So my answer is a resounding no, I will not be adding alcohol to my diet again. Suggesting skinny drinks alludes to my choice of maintaining my weight. While in the beginning my focus was in getting the weight off, it has evolved to health and wellness, not a scale.

I do not miss alcohol, and I have learned to enjoy my authentic, unaltered self. I like to be present in all situations, whether a nature hike, or a pub with friends. I don't mind if others partake around me, but I do prefer to avoid being around when others are overindulging. At those times, I will excuse myself and go do the things that I enjoy. I am aware of my limits and I respect them.

Wait, I thought cirrhosis could not be healed?

Someone in one of my support groups chastised me for sharing my story of reversal. They imply that by doing so I was disrespecting those who struggle and die from the condition, and I am giving them false hope. Others have heard that while you can reverse fatty liver and certain levels of fibrosis, once it's cirrhosis you cannot reverse it. First, know that I am not here to do any such thing; the opposite is true. I wish to offer hope that we can achieve our best, healthiest selves even if that means freezing our health in place or partial recovery. Second, studies now show that reversal is possible in certain cases, which I have shared earlier in this book. No matter how severe our condition may be, learning to care for ourselves helps the body, mind, and heart.

Making changes takes effort. Nobody can feed us every morsel of what we need to heal. We must be willing to put in the work, get to know our bodies, fight for our health, and self-advocate. Like anything in life, you only get back what you're willing to put in, and if your heart and soul have anything to say about it, you'll get something good back. You must be patient — it's a life change.

Susan R. Pryde

Transformation

My butterfly visit back in October 2021 had me stuck on the theme of transformation. Wasn't all healing a form of this? Something went wrong, and we needed a change to right it. Would it be the same as before? Or would it be a little weaker? Or maybe, just maybe it could be better, stronger, faster (ok, shameless Bionic Man reference here). Often, when I had put some effort into bettering myself in the past, I would revert to my old ways. Over and over I resolved to eat better, move more, and practice self-care. I would do this for several months, begin to feel success, then poof, I didn't want to continue. It was too difficult, it was not convenient, or I was too busy. I had every excuse in the book, living in an endless cycle of coming close to my ultimate goal, only to let go and give up. Looking back, I know I needed to address the big picture. Why was I not worthy of my own self-care? What was stopping me from achieving my best self?

I recall reading a quote about the transformation of a caterpillar into a butterfly. If we disturb the caterpillar in the chrysalis during its transformation, it can cause it to fail. It is the struggle itself to re-emerge that builds the strength in its wings required to take flight. We need to experience the struggle to rise.[84] Now, I'm not saying: "hey guys! Leave me lying on the floor in a puddle if I fall down". I'll take your offered hand, kind words, or well wishes. The diagnosis of cirrhosis was a catalyst for some extraordinary changes in my life. It startled me into motion. The shock inspired me to say, "move along, folks, there's nothing more to see here" leading me to a new and healthier path.

---

[84] [84]Ferris Jabr, "How Does a Caterpillar Turn into a Butterfly?," Scientific American, accessed March 9, 2023, https://www.scientificamerican.com/article/caterpillar-butterfly-metamorphosis-explainer/.

What specifically has changed? I now start each day in the wee, dark hours all alone, soaking up information. I read websites about liver health, buy books on poetry and self-help. I study nutritional websites, and communicate in support groups. I take time to sit, eyes closed, and breathe. I started writing a blog, journaling how I was feeling, and what I was learning. I created a Facebook page titled "Living Well with Cirrhosis – Sue Pryde's Journey" and invited friends to join. I was seeking support and looking for people that might be feeling what I was feeling, and who needed help healing their bodies and hearts. I would share all I learned within my blog, encouraged now to keep reading and keep sharing my thoughts. I shared my positive progress in support groups, and others began to ask me how I achieved my success. Often, I responded by pointing them to my blog and my platform started growing. I realized that my words were of comfort to others, and it drove me to keep learning and growing. I had a purpose to not only help myself, but others would benefit, too. I was growing a group of people to work together and heal with! This was amazing to me.

Early on, everything was scary, heavy, and dark, but over time my world has become an enlightening, nourishing place full of light. Broken parts I ignored are now healing. My body is changing for the better. I am healing and regenerating those parts that are willing and able. My mind, spirit, and soul are all benefiting from the growth. I now seek the little things in life, feel more joy and have more curiosity in learning how things fit together. I'm wondering why, in my youth, I did not pay more attention to poets, philosophers, and nourishment.

Susan R. Pryde

Don't be afraid to transform, my friends. This time, when standing over that threshold of change, I closed my eyes and took the next step, rather than rolling back down the hill. I can tell you it's a beautiful sight to behold, and worth staying the course. I let my transformation unfold, and I will continue to do so.

Conclusion

Congratulations! You have made your first decision to heal by reading my book. I desire for you an uphill climb and a renewed sense of confidence to succeed. What will YOUR next step be?

I wrote the book that I longed for when I first learned that I had liver disease. I could not find what I needed in any one source, which drove me to make sure something was available for others. I hope you have found comfort and information to help you move forward. Here are some tips:

- Build a solid support team of friends and family, and let others help you
- Find the right doctors who respond, inform, and care about your progress. Ask them questions and follow through
- Seek specialists if you need them. If you don't know how to eat healthily, go to a nutritionist. If you are hurting mentally, get a psychologist. If you need help with substance abuse, go for counseling
- Join support groups in person or online
- Learn what makes you happy and go do it
- Practice proper self-care
- Allow yourself to feel emotions in a healthy way
- Learn to take good care of your whole being. Take the time to address each aspect in your own fashion and do what feels right

Susan R. Pryde

I would love to see you on my website, blog, private support group, or Instagram. Or, feel free to send me an e-mail.

- Website: https://susanpryde.wixsite.com/website
- Facebook blog: "Living Well with Cirrhosis – Sue Pryde's Journey"
- Facebook private support group: "Living Well with Cirrhosis – One Liver at a Time"
- Instagram: https://www.instagram.com/healprydeliver/
- E-mail: healprydeliver@gmail.com

Heal well and let me know how you're doing! I honestly want to know.

Love, Sue

References

"5 Essential Questions and 10 Tips to Create Positive
Change | Psychology Today." Accessed March 9,
2023.
https://www.psychologytoday.com/us/blog/the-
integrationist/201405/5-essential-questions-and-
10-tips-create-positive-change.

"5 Mindful Steps for Self-Observation | Psychology Today."
Accessed March 9, 2023.
https://www.psychologytoday.com/us/blog/mindf
ul-recovery/202109/5-mindful-steps-self-
observation.

"14 Self-Care Rituals to Practice Now | Psychology Today."
Accessed March 18, 2023.
https://www.psychologytoday.com/us/blog/the-
empowerment-diary/202207/14-self-care-rituals-
practice-now.

"A Good Guide to Good Carbs: The Glycemic Index -
Harvard Health." Accessed March 9, 2023.
https://www.health.harvard.edu/healthbeat/a-
good-guide-to-good-carbs-the-glycemic-index.

Alves-Bezerra, Michele, and David E. Cohen. "Triglyceride
Metabolism in the Liver." *Comprehensive
Physiology* 8, no. 1 (December 12, 2017): 1.
https://doi.org/10.1002/cphy.c170012.

Ask the Experts: Acute and Sudden Liver Failure. Accessed
March 9, 2023.
https://www.youtube.com/watch?v=aleXOXHSO_s
.

Associates in Gastroenterology. "What Is Fibroscan |
Testing Preparation & Expectations." Accessed
March 9, 2023.
https://agcosprings.com/procedures/fibroscan/.

Atkinson, Fiona S., Kaye Foster-Powell, and Jennie C.
Brand-Miller. "International Tables of Glycemic
Index and Glycemic Load Values: 2008." *Diabetes*

Susan R. Pryde

Care 31, no. 12 (December 2008): 2281.
https://doi.org/10.2337/dc08-1239.

Bikeyeva, Viktoriya, Ahmed Abdullah, Aleksandra
Radivojevic, Anas A. Abu Jad, Anvesh Ravanavena,
Chetna Ravindra, Emmanuelar O. Igweonu-
Nwakile, et al. "Nonalcoholic Fatty Liver Disease
and Hypothyroidism: What You Need to Know."
Cureus 14, no. 8 (August 2022).
https://doi.org/10.7759/cureus.28052.

Carneiro, Carolina, Jorge Brito, Carlos Bilreiro, Marta
Barros, Carla Bahia, Inês Santiago, and Filipe
Caseiro-Alves. "All about Portal Vein: A Pictorial
Display to Anatomy, Variants and
Physiopathology." *Insights into Imaging* 10
(December 2019). https://doi.org/10.1186/s13244-
019-0716-8.

"Chronic Illness and Ambiguous Loss | Psychology Today."
Accessed March 9, 2023.
https://www.psychologytoday.com/us/blog/chroni
cally-me/202103/chronic-illness-and-ambiguous-
loss.

"Cirrhosis (Severe Scarring) - American Liver Foundation,"
June 9, 2022. https://liverfoundation.org/about-
your-liver/how-liver-diseases-progress/cirrhosis-
severe-scarring/.

Cleveland Clinic. "CPAP Machine: What It Is, How It Works,
Pros & Cons." Accessed March 9, 2023.
https://my.clevelandclinic.org/health/treatments/2
2043-cpap-machine.

"Doctor Dolittle - Wikipedia." Accessed March 9, 2023.
https://en.wikipedia.org/wiki/Doctor_Dolittle.

Dreams, Superstitions, Symbolic Meanings Guide. "You
Searched for Orange and Black Butterfly," May 28,
2021. https://blogoguide.com/search/orange and
black butterfly/.

E, Piantanida, Ippolito S, Gallo D, Masiello E, Premoli P, Cusini C, Rosetti S, et al. "The Interplay between Thyroid and Liver: Implications for Clinical Practice." *Journal of Endocrinological Investigation* 43, no. 7 (July 2020). https://doi.org/10.1007/s40618-020-01208-6.

"Elevated Liver Enzymes - Mayo Clinic." Accessed May 15, 2023. https://www.mayoclinic.org/symptoms/elevated-liver-enzymes/basics/definition/sym-20050830.

"End Stage Liver Disease - American Liver Foundation," June 13, 2022. https://liverfoundation.org/about-your-liver/how-liver-diseases-progress/end-stage-liver-disease/.

"Fast-Food Fans May Face Liver Damage." Accessed March 9, 2023. https://www.webmd.com/diet/news/20230113/fast-food-fans-may-face-liver-damage.

"Fibrosis (Scarring) - American Liver Foundation," June 9, 2022. https://liverfoundation.org/about-your-liver/how-liver-diseases-progress/fibrosis-scarring/.

"Frontiers | Potential Effects of Coronaviruses on the Liver: An Update." Accessed March 9, 2023. https://www.frontiersin.org/articles/10.3389/fmed.2021.651658/full.

GIS. "Your Liver & Cirrhosis Poster." *Gastrointestinal Society* (blog). Accessed March 14, 2023. https://badgut.org/information-centre/multimedia/your-liver-cirrhosis/.

"Glycemic Index – Glycemic Index Research and GI News." Accessed March 9, 2023. https://glycemicindex.com/.

"Heal by Connecting with Others | Psychology Today." Accessed March 9, 2023. https://www.psychologytoday.com/us/blog/anxiet

y-another-name-pain/202205/heal-connecting-
others.

"Hepatocellular Carcinoma: 5 Things to Know." Accessed
May 15, 2023.
https://www.medscape.com/viewarticle/925146.

"High-Salt Diet May Harm Liver," February 25, 2016.
https://www.medicalnewstoday.com/articles/3070
28.

J, Zheng, Hoffman Kl, Chen Js, Shivappa N, Sood A,
Browman Gj, Dirba Dd, et al. "Dietary Inflammatory
Potential in Relation to the Gut Microbiome:
Results from a Cross-Sectional Study." *The British
Journal of Nutrition* 124, no. 9 (November 14,
2020).
https://doi.org/10.1017/S0007114520001853.

Jabr, Ferris. "How Does a Caterpillar Turn into a Butterfly?"
Scientific American. Accessed March 9, 2023.
https://www.scientificamerican.com/article/caterp
illar-butterfly-metamorphosis-explainer/.

Kalaitzakis, Evangelos. "Gastrointestinal Dysfunction in
Liver Cirrhosis." *World Journal of
Gastroenterology : WJG* 20, no. 40 (October 10,
2014): 14686.
https://doi.org/10.3748/wjg.v20.i40.14686.

"KonMari Method: Life-Changing Online Tidying Course."
Accessed March 9, 2023.
https://learn.konmari.com/?campaign=ShfyNav.

Kota, Sunil Kumar, Lalit Kumar Meher, S. V. S. Krishna, and
K. D. Modi. "Hypothyroidism in Metabolic
Syndrome." *Indian Journal of Endocrinology and
Metabolism* 16, no. Suppl 2 (December 2012):
S332. https://doi.org/10.4103/2230-8210.104079.

"Learning to Live Well with Chronic Illness/Conditions |
Psychology Today." Accessed March 18, 2023.
https://www.psychologytoday.com/us/blog/some-

assembly-required/201601/learning-live-well-
chronic-illnessconditions.

"Levothyroxine (Oral Route) Description and Brand Names
- Mayo Clinic." Accessed March 9, 2023.
https://www.mayoclinic.org/drugs-
supplements/levothyroxine-oral-
route/description/drg-20072133.

"Liver Cancer - American Liver Foundation," June 9, 2022.
https://liverfoundation.org/about-your-liver/how-
liver-diseases-progress/liver-cancer/.

"Liver Disease Diets: Fatty Liver Diet and More," June 15,
2022. https://liverfoundation.org/health-and-
wellness/healthy-lifestyle/liver-disease-diets/.

LIVESTRONG.COM. "Benefits of Turmeric Powder."
Accessed March 9, 2023.
https://www.livestrong.com/article/145900-
benefits-of-turmeric-powder/.

LIVESTRONG.COM. "Cottage Cheese and Digestion."
Accessed March 9, 2023.
https://www.livestrong.com/article/502258-
cottage-cheese-and-digestion/.

LIVESTRONG.COM. "Dizziness & Nausea When Losing
Weight Too Fast." Accessed March 9, 2023.
https://www.livestrong.com/article/425420-
dizziness-nausea-losing-weight-fast/.

LIVESTRONG.COM. "How Does the Food We Eat Actually
Give Us Energy?" Accessed March 9, 2023.
https://www.livestrong.com/article/444740-how-
does-the-food-we-eat-actually-give-us-energy/.

LIVESTRONG.COM. "Instead of Cutting Carbs, Choose The
Right Ones With This Guide." Accessed March 9,
2023. https://www.livestrong.com/article/35816-
list-good-bad-carbs/.

LIVESTRONG.COM. "Is a Teaspoon of Ground Cinnamon
Good for You?" Accessed March 9, 2023.

Susan R. Pryde

https://www.livestrong.com/article/495786-is-a-teaspoon-of-ground-cinnamon-good-for-you/.

LIVESTRONG.COM. "Nutritional Value of Blackberries & Blueberries." Accessed March 9, 2023. https://www.livestrong.com/article/527147-nutritional-value-of-blackberries-blueberries/.

LIVESTRONG.COM. "The Dosage of Ground Flaxseed." Accessed March 9, 2023. https://www.livestrong.com/article/456688-the-dosage-of-ground-flaxseed/.

LIVESTRONG.COM. "The Fascinating Link Between Walnuts and Weight Loss." Accessed March 9, 2023. https://www.livestrong.com/article/13559046-walnuts-could-hold-the-key-to-weight-loss/.

LIVESTRONG.COM. "What Is Metabolic Syndrome, Exactly?" Accessed March 9, 2023. https://www.livestrong.com/article/13723809-metabolic-syndrome/.

LIVESTRONG.COM. "Why Are Beets Good for You?" Accessed March 9, 2023. https://www.livestrong.com/article/413049-why-are-beets-good-for-you/.

May 14, WAYNE ESKRIDGE | 573 40sc and 2018. "Can Cirrhosis Be Reversed? Of Course Not They Say, but What If." Fatty Liver Foundation. Accessed May 16, 2023. https://www.fattyliverfoundation.org/reverse_cirrhosis.

Mayo Clinic. "Blood Pressure Chart: What Your Reading Means." Accessed June 29, 2023. https://www.mayoclinic.org/diseases-conditions/high-blood-pressure/in-depth/blood-pressure/art-20050982.

Mayo Clinic. "Cirrhosis FAQs." Accessed March 9, 2023. https://www.mayoclinic.org/diseases-conditions/cirrhosis/multimedia/vid-20532300.

Mayo Clinic. "Esophageal Varices - Symptoms and Causes." Accessed March 9, 2023. https://www.mayoclinic.org/diseases-conditions/esophageal-varices/symptoms-causes/syc-20351538.

Mayo Clinic. "Hyponatremia - Symptoms and Causes." Accessed March 9, 2023. https://www.mayoclinic.org/diseases-conditions/hyponatremia/symptoms-causes/syc-20373711.

Mayo Clinic. "Nonalcoholic Fatty Liver Disease - Symptoms and Causes." Accessed March 9, 2023. https://www.mayoclinic.org/diseases-conditions/nonalcoholic-fatty-liver-disease/symptoms-causes/syc-20354567.

Miedaner, Talane. "3 Laws of Attraction: Start with the Present Is Always Perfect." *LifeCoach.Com* (blog), February 25, 2015. https://www.lifecoach.com/articles/laws-of-attraction/3-laws-attraction-the-present-is-always-perfect/.

"Nonalcoholic Fatty Liver Disease (NAFLD) - American Liver Foundation," May 23, 2022. https://liverfoundation.org/liver-diseases/fatty-liver-disease/nonalcoholic-fatty-liver-disease-nafld/.

Noom, Inc. "Noom: Stop Dieting. Get Life-Long Results." Accessed March 9, 2023. https://www.noom.com.

Print, Mayo Clinic Staff. "Liver Problems - Alternative Medicine." Mayo Clinic. Accessed May 20, 2023. https://www.mayoclinic.org/diseases-conditions/liver-problems/diagnosis-treatment/alternative-medicine/scc-20374505.

Putnam, Rose. "What Is The Spiritual Meaning Of a Butterfly Landing On You?" *Crystal Clear Intuition* (blog). Accessed March 9, 2023.

Susan R. Pryde

> https://crystalclearintuition.com/butterfly-landing-on-you-spiritual/.

Saitz, Richard. "Introduction to Alcohol Withdrawal." *Alcohol Health and Research World* 22, no. 1 (1998): 5.

Simpson, Rachel F., Carol Hermon, Bette Liu, Jane Green, Gillian K. Reeves, Valerie Beral, and Sarah Floud. "Alcohol Drinking Patterns and Liver Cirrhosis Risk: Analysis of the Prospective UK Million Women Study." *The Lancet Public Health* 4, no. 1 (January 1, 2019): e41–48. https://doi.org/10.1016/S2468-2667(18)30230-5.

"Skinny Liver: A Proven Program to Prevent and Reverse the New Silent Epidemic-Fatty Liver Disease: Kirkpatrick MS RD LD, Kristin, Hanouneh MD, Ibrahim: 9780738219165: Amazon.Com: Books." Accessed March 9, 2023. https://www.amazon.com/Skinny-Liver-Program-Prevent-Epidemic/dp/0738219169.

STUDIO TENN TALKS: SHAUN CASSIDY & PATRICK CASSIDY, 2021. https://www.youtube.com/watch?v=yFy5PlGYrbE.

"The Alcoholic Liver Disease/Nonalcoholic Fatty Liver Disease Index (ANI) - Medical Professionals - Mayo Clinic." Accessed March 9, 2023. https://www.mayoclinic.org/medical-professionals/transplant-medicine/calculators/the-alcoholic-liver-disease-nonalcoholic-fatty-liver-disease-index-ani/itt-20434726.

"The Healthy Liver - American Liver Foundation," June 9, 2022. https://liverfoundation.org/about-your-liver/how-liver-diseases-progress/the-healthy-liver/.

"The Power of Letting Go | Psychology Today." Accessed March 9, 2023.

https://www.psychologytoday.com/us/blog/test-case/201203/the-power-letting-go.

"The Stages of Liver Disease - American Liver Foundation," June 8, 2022. https://liverfoundation.org/about-your-liver/how-liver-diseases-progress/.

This Naked Mind. "Annie Grace." Accessed March 9, 2023. https://thisnakedmind.com/.

"Understanding Your Liver Elastography (FibroScan®) Results | Memorial Sloan Kettering Cancer Center." Accessed March 9, 2023. https://www.mskcc.org/cancer-care/patient-education/understanding-your-fibroscan-results.

"Unexpected Joy – Just Another WordPress Site." Accessed March 9, 2023. https://unexpectedjoy.co.uk/.

"Upper Endoscopy - Mayo Clinic." Accessed March 9, 2023. https://www.mayoclinic.org/tests-procedures/endoscopy/about/pac-20395197.

"Vasovagal Syncope - Diagnosis and Treatment - Mayo Clinic." Accessed March 9, 2023. https://www.mayoclinic.org/diseases-conditions/vasovagal-syncope/diagnosis-treatment/drc-20350531.

Weiss, Cynthia. "Mayo Clinic Q and A: 10 Nutrition Myths Debunked." Mayo Clinic News Network, July 31, 2022. https://newsnetwork.mayoclinic.org/discussion/mayo-clinic-q-and-a-10-nutrition-myths-debunked/.

"What Does Emotional Medical Trauma Look Like? | Psychology Today." Accessed March 18, 2023. https://www.psychologytoday.com/us/blog/afraid-the-doctor/202206/what-does-emotional-medical-trauma-look.

"Where Your Mind Meets Your Body | Psychology Today." Accessed March 9, 2023. https://www.psychologytoday.com/us/blog/your-

Susan R. Pryde

brain-on-body-dysmorphia/202211/where-your-mind-meets-your-body.

Yadav, Anitha, and Elizabeth J. Carey. "Osteoporosis in Chronic Liver Disease." *Nutrition in Clinical Practice* 28, no. 1 (February 1, 2013): 52–64. https://doi.org/10.1177/0884533612470145.

"You Have to Feel to Heal: Emotional Awareness | Psychology Today." Accessed March 9, 2023. https://www.psychologytoday.com/us/blog/anxiety-another-name-pain/202112/you-have-feel-heal-emotional-awareness.

"Your Body's Reaction To Yo-Yo Diets Explained." Accessed March 9, 2023. https://www.webmd.com/diet/ss/slideshow-diet-yo-yo-diet-effect.